Eat to Beat High Blood Pressure

£13

Eat to Beat High Blood Pressure

Natural Self-help for Hypertension, including 60 recipes

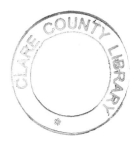

Dr Sarah Brewer *and*
Michelle Berriedale-Johnson

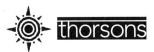

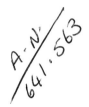

Thorsons
An Imprint of HarperCollins*Publishers*
77–85 Fulham Palace Road
Hammersmith, London W6 8JB

The website address is: www.thorsonselement.com

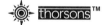™

and *Thorsons* are trademarks of
HarperCollins*Publishers* Ltd

Published by Thorsons 2003

10 9 8 7 6

© Dr Sarah Brewer and Michelle Berriedale-Johnson 2003

Dr Sarah Brewer and Michelle Berriedale-Johnson assert the moral right to be
identified as the authors of this work

A catalogue record for this book is
available from the British Library

ISBN-13 978-0-00-714135-7
ISBN-10 0-00-714135-1

Printed and bound in Great Britain by
Martins the Printers, Berwick upon Tweed

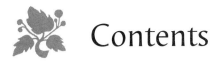

Contents

Introduction

Whether or not you develop high blood pressure (hypertension) is influenced by several factors. These are your genes, the way you eat, and other aspects of your lifestyle such as the amount of exercise you take, whether or not you smoke, and the amount of alcohol you drink. Eating to beat high blood pressure is not only possible, it is one of the mainstays of effective treatment. This book looks at how various dietary changes can help to reduce a raised blood pressure and lessen your risk of developing associated complications such as coronary heart disease and stroke.

Making simple, healthy changes to your lifestyle can also significantly reduce your chances of contracting coronary heart disease. For instance, if you stop smoking, your risk of getting heart disease drops by 50–70 per cent within five years. If you take up regular exercise, your risk falls by 45 per cent. Keeping your alcohol intake within healthy limits will also have a beneficial effect. Drinking two or three units a day can reduce your chances of heart disease by as much as 25–45 per cent, but excessive intakes increase the risk. Losing excess body weight will bring your chances of heart disease down by 35–55 per cent. For more on lifestyle changes, see Chapters 20 and 21.

Food supplements are also effective in helping to maintain a healthy circulation. For more about these, please see Chapter 19.

The delicious recipes provided by Michelle Berriedale-Johnson will make eating to beat hypertension as pleasant and easy as possible.

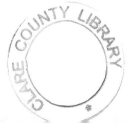

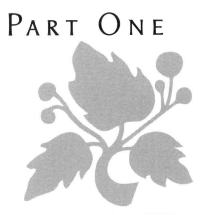

PART ONE

The Facts about High Blood Pressure

CHAPTER 1

What is High Blood Pressure?

Everyone needs a certain blood pressure (BP) to keep blood moving around their body and maintain their circulation. Blood pressure exists because your heart pumps blood around a closed system, rather like a boiler pumping water through a series of central heating pipes. The pressure in your arteries therefore depends on a number of factors, including the volume of fluid inside your circulation, how hard your heart is pumping at any given time, and the elasticity or 'resistance' of the vessels the blood is passing through.

Normal BP varies naturally throughout the day and night, going up and down in response to your emotions and level of activity. If you have high blood pressure, however, your BP will remain consistently high, even when you are asleep.

The heart alternately contracts and relaxes as it pumps to produce the heartbeat. Each contraction produces a surge in pressure. The highest pressure reached in the arteries during this surge is known as the *systolic* pressure as it is due to contraction (systole) of the heart. As the heart rests between beats, blood pressure falls again and the lowest blood pressure recorded while the heart rests (diastole) is known as the *diastolic* pressure. In general, as the heart pumps more strongly, systolic pressure rises, while a reduction in elasticity of the peripheral arteries causes diastolic pressure to go up.

How BP is Measured

Blood pressure (BP) is measured using an instrument called a sphygmomanometer. This has an inflatable cuff which goes around your upper arm, a small pump to push air into the cuff and a column of mercury (or a dial) to record the pressure within the cuff.

As the cuff is inflated with air, the person measuring your BP usually feels for a pulse (brachial artery) in the crook of your elbow. While the pressure within your artery stays higher than that in the cuff, blood can be felt pulsing through. Once the pressure in the cuff becomes greater than that in your artery, the vessel is squashed flat and blood stops flowing through it at that point. By inflating the cuff to an initial pressure that is higher than the expected systolic pressure, then listening with a stethoscope over your brachial artery as the pressure is slowly released, the point at which blood manages to squirt through again with each pulse can be heard distinctly as a tapping sound. The pressure registering in the cuff at this point is taken as your systolic BP. The cuff is then slowly deflated further while listening over your artery. The tapping sounds become louder, then change to a dull whooshing noise before disappearing. The point at which blood can no longer be heard whooshing through the vessel is taken as your diastolic BP. The pulsing noise heard in the artery between these two pressures is a result of turbulence as the cuff impinges on the vessel and deforms its walls. We therefore know that the blood pressure in the artery is the same as that in the cuff at the point where the sounds disappear, as turbulence is no longer occurring. BP can also be measured with modern digital cuffs that fit around the wrist.

BP is measured according to the length of a column of mercury it can support. It is therefore expressed in millimetres of mercury (mmHg). BP is written down as the higher pressure (systole) over the lower figure (diastole).

* A typical 20-year-old may have a BP of around 120/70 mmHg.
* BP naturally tends to rise with age and a fit 50-year-old may have a BP of around 135/85 mmHg.
* The pulse pressure – the difference between the systolic and diastolic pressures – is normally around 50 mmHg.
* If your BP is consistently higher than 140/90, then you are suffering from high blood pressure, or hypertension.

How Blood Pressure is Controlled

Blood pressure is normally controlled and kept within safe limits by the body in a number of ways, including:

* changing the rate at which the heart pumps
* widening or constricting small arteries
* altering the amount of blood pooled in the veins
* varying the amount of salt and fluids filtered from the circulation via the kidneys.

These factors are controlled by nerve signals from the brain, and by several different hormones. As a result, normal BP varies naturally throughout the day, going up and down in response to your emotions and level of activity. It is lowest during sleep (usually at around 3am) and highest in the morning from just before you wake until around 11 am. If you have high blood pressure, however, your BP will remain high all the time, even at rest.

Hypertension

As many as one in five adults have high blood pressure, known medically as hypertension. This means that blood is forced through their system under a constantly high pressure. Hypertension is diagnosed when systolic pressure is consistently greater than 140 mmHg and diastolic pressure consistently greater than 90 mmHg. A systolic blood pressure between 140–160 mmHg and diastolic values between 90–95 mmHg are sometimes referred to as mild hypertension.

In hypertension, the body's systems for correcting high or low blood pressure don't seem to work properly so blood pressure is maintained at an elevated level compared to normal. Little is known about how or why this happens, but the condition seems to be readily reversible once diet and lifestyle changes are introduced, together with any necessary anti-hypertensive drug treatment.

SYMPTOMS

Unfortunately, people with high blood pressure usually notice very little in the way of symptoms, although a few may develop a pounding sensation in their ears or a splitting headache. As a result, hypertension is often referred to as the silent killer, as it usually creeps up on you without any obvious warning. Even if your blood pressure is dangerously high, you may feel relatively well. If symptoms do occur, they tend to be non-specific, such as a headache or getting up at night to pass urine more often than normal. Your blood pressure has to be severely raised before you develop dizziness or visual disturbances. It is therefore a good idea for adults to have their blood pressure checked on a regular basis, every year or so – especially if high blood pressure runs in their family. This is because a high blood pressure that remains undiagnosed and untreated can lead to a number of potentially serious complications.

WHY HIGH BLOOD PRESSURE IS HARMFUL

Hypertension is not a disease in itself, but a clinical sign that you are at increased risk of a number of serious health problems. As blood is forced through your system at high pressure, your artery walls receive a pounding. This which can both over-stretch important blood vessels as well as damage their linings. If left untreated, this can trigger premature hardening and furring up of the arteries (atherosclerosis) and increase the risk of a number of health problems. If your blood pressure remains constantly high, this can lead to:

* peripheral vascular disease – when arteries supplying blood to the limbs become hardened and furred up so circulation is reduced
* impotence – when the blood supply to the penis is affected
* failing sight – when blood vessels in the eyes are affected
* kidney failure – when blood vessels in your kidneys are damaged
* heart failure – when your heart finds it difficult to pump blood against the high pressure in your circulation; this typically causes breathlessness as fluid builds up in your lungs
* angina (heart pain) – when the excess workload on the heart increases its oxygen and nutrient needs beyond those provided by its blood supply
* a heart attack – when the coronary arteries are damaged enough to trigger a sudden blockage of blood supply to the heart muscle (e.g. due to a blood clot)
* a stroke – when blood vessels in the brain are damaged enough to cause a disruption in blood supply to brain cells, – either due to a sudden blood clot, or to a haemorrhage.

Research shows that for a man in his 40s:

* each rise in systolic blood pressure of 10mmHg increases his risk of heart disease by 20 per cent
* the risk of having a stroke is 30 times higher if he has high blood pressure than for someone with normal BP.

This all sounds rather frightening, but the good news is that early diagnosis and treatment can control your blood pressure and keep you healthy. It is vitally important that your hypertension is well controlled, by taking your tablets exactly as prescribed. A number of relatively simple dietary and lifestyle changes can also help to reduce the risk of high blood pressure, lower a BP that is already raised and reduce the risk of complications such as coronary heart disease. If these changes were to reduce your diastolic BP by as little as 5 mmHg, they would decrease your risk of coronary heart disease by 16 per cent, and if they succeeded in reducing your average blood pressure by 10 mmHg, this would reduce your risk of premature death by as much as a third. You really can eat to beat the unwanted effects of high blood pressure.

UNDIAGNOSED HYPERTENSION

Ideally, all adults should have their blood pressure measured regularly, at least once every three years, or more often as your doctor recommends. If your blood pressure is found to be high, you will have it measured several times before your doctor decides whether or not to prescribe any anti-hypertensive drugs. This is to make sure your blood pressure remains consistently high and is not just going up as a result of visiting the surgery. Once you start taking blood pressure treatment, you may be on it for life – but you will probably live longer as a result.

Unfortunately, an estimated one in two people with high blood pressure are undiagnosed, and of those that are picked up and treated, at least another half do not have acceptable blood pressure control. This is mostly because the condition rarely makes you feel ill, and having to take one, two or even three tablets per day to treat something that is not an illness, but a risk factor for other diseases, is understandably frustrating. However, early diagnosis and successful treatment of high blood pressure is vital for continued long-term health.

Types of High Blood Pressure

Ninety per cent of people with high blood pressure, have no obvious single cause and are said to have *primary*, or *essential*, *hypertension*. The remaining one in ten people with high blood pressure have an identifiable underlying factor, such as kidney problems, a hormone imbalance or drug side-effects, and are said to have *secondary hypertension*.

Malignant hypertension refers to the most dangerous type of high blood pressure in which pressures go very high, often very quickly. This can damage internal organs over a short period of time and is sometimes also referred to as *accelerated hypertension*. It is treated as a medical emergency because if diastolic pressure remains above 120 mmHg for a prolonged period of time, the linings of small blood vessels (arterioles) are damaged and start to leak. When looked at under the microscope, the blood vessel walls have literally started to crumble (*fibrinoid necrosis*). This lets protein-rich fluid, and sometimes whole blood, seep out of the blood stream to build up in the tissues. As well as interfering with blood supply to that part of the body, the leakages cause damage, inflammation and scarring – commonly to the kidneys, backs of the eyes and in the brain. This is known as *target organ damage*. Damage to the kidneys also results in the release of hormones that put the blood pressure up even more, so a vicious cycle builds up. Treatment aims to bring BP down slowly over several days so that the body can adjust to lower pressures again.

To differentiate it from malignant hypertension, primary high blood pressure is often referred to as *benign essential hypertension.*

Refractory hypertension refers to high blood pressure that does not respond to standard first-line anti-hypertensive drug treatments. Although this is uncommon, referral to a specialist is needed so that investigations and treatment with other drugs can be started.

CHAPTER 2

Causes, Diagnosis and Treatment of High Blood Pressure

Blood pressure naturally tends to rise with age, so that high blood pressure is more common in middle life and beyond. Some people, especially males, may develop it in their 20s or even earlier, however. Blood pressure is also known to vary with race – those of African origin tend to have higher blood pressures than Caucasians, for example.

Causes of Essential Hypertension

Several factors are thought to be involved in the development of primary, or benign essential hypertension. These include inherited factors (high blood pressure runs in some families), developmental factors (occurring during embryonic life in the womb) and environmental factors such as diet and lifestyle, which you can address to help lower a high blood pressure.

INHERITED FACTORS

Essential hypertension is thought to result from inherited genes that may trigger high blood pressure as a result of one or more abnormalities involving:

* sensitivity of the blood pressure monitors (baroreceptors) throughout the circulation
* altered secretion of, or sensitivity to, hormones (e.g. anti-diuretic hormone, renin, aldosterone) or other chemicals that help to regulate normal blood pressure
* dilation or constriction of blood vessels in response to pressure changes
* nerve control of BP or abnormal signals from the brain
* control of the amount of fluid and salt in the circulation
* control of the strength and rate of the heartbeat.

Researchers have already identified a gene that may be able to predict your future risk of hypertension. People who have inherited the angiotensinogen gene (T235) from both parents have double the risk of developing high blood pressure and coronary heart disease compared to those who do not have the gene variant, or who inherit it only from one parent.

DEVELOPMENTAL FACTORS

Fascinating research has suggests the way you develop during the first few weeks of life as an embryo may affect your future risk of high blood pressure and other cardiovascular diseases in adult life. This is probably linked with lack of micronutrients (vitamin and minerals) in the mother's diet, which affects the way your arteries are laid down. Researchers have found, for example, that:

* Low birth-weight babies maybe more likely to develop high blood pressure as adults. Average adult systolic BP increases by 11 mmHg as birth weight goes down from 7.5lb to 5.5lb.
* The size of the placenta may be important – average systolic blood pressure rises by 15 mmHg as placental weight increases from 1lb to 1.5lb .
* The highest blood pressures occur in men and women who were born as small babies with large placentas.
* Risk of high blood pressure in later life also increases:
    - as a baby's birth length decreases
    - as the ratio of a baby's head circumference to the length of the baby increases from less than 0.65 to 0.7 or more.
    - if the mother's blood haemoglobin level was low during pregnancy
    - if maternal nutrition was known to be poor.

Lack of important nutrients – including vitamins, minerals and essential fatty acids – during the first few weeks of embryonic life is thought to trigger the development of abnormal arterial and blood circulatory patterns. These probably result from an imbalance between the placenta and baby. This is supported by research linking fingerprint patterns with the risk of developing high blood pressure in later life. Fingerprints are laid down in the womb in the first few weeks following conception. Their patterns are linked to the degree of bumpiness and swelling of the developing fingertips, which is related in turn to irregular blood circulation.

Fingerprint patterns take the form of arches, loops or whorls, and the more whorls you have, the more likely you are to become hypertensive in later life. People with at least one whorl may have a blood pressure that is 6 per cent higher (8mmHg) than people with no whorls. BP then generally increases as the number of whorls increases, up to the maximum number possible, which is ten (two per digit). The average number tends to be two or three. Long, narrow hands are also associated with higher blood pressure, and both effects are more marked on the right hand.

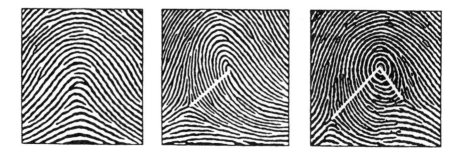

Inherited and developmental factors are not the sole causes of high blood pressure, however. Something else has to happen in any individual before blood pressure goes up, and this is where environmental factors come in. These interact with inherited factors in individuals whose genes predispose them to hypertension to produce high blood pressure in later life. If several environmental factors linked with high blood pressure interact together, your risk of high blood pressure will be even greater.

ATHEROSCLEROSIS

One of the main causes of high blood pressure – especially a raised systolic BP – is hardening, furring up and narrowing of the arteries (atherosclerosis – *see Chapter 3*). This occurs naturally with increasing age and comes on more quickly if you smoke, eat an excessively fatty diet or are overweight. High blood pressure in turn puts excessive strain on the arterial wall lining and triggers damage that hastens atherosclerosis. Because atherosclerosis in turn causes hardening of arterial walls, a vicious cycle is set up in which blood vessels become even less elastic and less able to distend to even out pressure surges, so BP rises further. High blood pressure is therefore both a cause, and a consequence, of atherosclerosis, with each factor making the other worse.

DIABETES

Diabetes mellitus is a condition in which blood sugar (glucose) levels are raised due to insufficient production of insulin hormone by the pancreas. Some people also have an impaired tolerance to glucose tolerance due to an inability of their cells to respond properly to relatively normal levels of insulin (insulin resistance). Having poorly controlled diabetes significantly increases the risk of developing atherosclerosis, high blood pressure, coronary heart disease (CHD) and stroke – especially in women. The reason is not fully understood, but high blood sugar levels may trigger abnormal blood clotting, damage blood vessel linings to trigger hardening and furring up, affect nerves controlling heart and blood vessel function or weaken muscles in the heart or artery walls.

The risk of severe CHD is two to three times higher in men with diabetes and three to seven times higher in women with diabetes. Therefore, if you have both high blood pressure and are also diabetic, it is vitally important that you keep your blood sugar levels under tight control.

SMOKING

Smoking cigarettes greatly increases the risks associated with hypertension – people with high blood pressure, who also smoke, are two or three times more likely to develop coronary heart disease than hypertensive non-smokers, and life-insurance companies load their premiums accordingly.

Smoking cigarettes triggers hardening and furring up of the arteries (atherosclerosis), which is one of the most important causes of high blood pressure, coronary heart disease and stroke. It is also linked with at least 90 per cent of all cancers. The reason that cigarette smoke is so toxic is that it contains chemicals that:

* damage the lining of arterial walls, triggering the build-up of clots and plaques
* increase the stickiness of blood, making serious blood clots (thrombosis) more likely
* displace oxygen from red blood cells in exchange for poisonous carbon monoxide – so that less

oxygen is available for use by cells, including those in the heart muscle and artery walls

✹ trigger spasm of arteries all over the body, which increases blood pressure and decreases blood flow to vital areas such as the brain and heart

✹ produce harmful by-products of metabolism known as free radicals which damage tissues, increasing the risk of atherosclerosis and also of cancer.

For more information, see Chapter 21.

OBESITY

People who are overweight or obese are more likely to have high blood pressure than thin people, as there is a larger body tissue mass through which the heart has to pump blood. Overweight people are also more likely to eat an unhealthy diet with a high intake of saturated fat. This raises blood fat levels, which in turn hastens the onset of atherosclerosis. Another factor is that overweight people tend to be inactive.

Although not everyone who is overweight has high blood pressure, however, there seems to be an interaction between obesity and some underlying, predisposing mechanism that is inherited by some people. This may be linked to where excess fat is stored. Overweight people who carry excess weight around their middle (apple-shaped) rather than around their hips (pear-shaped) seem to be at greater risk of a number of health conditions, including high blood pressure, atherosclerosis, raised cholesterol levels, diabetes, CHD and stroke. The reasons are not fully understood but may be linked to the way the body metabolizes dietary fats.

For more information, see Chapter 21.

ALCOHOL

A high alcohol intake is also linked with an increased risk of hypertension. People who regularly consume excessive amounts (more than 3 units of alcohol per day, or 21 units per week) tend to have higher blood pressures. However, many people drink more than this and have a normal blood pressure – it depends on whether you have inherited predisposing factors that make you sensitive to these effects of alcohol.

For more information, see Chapters 11 and 21.

LACK OF EXERCISE

Lack of exercise is an important cause of high blood pressure. Inactivity means the heart is unfit, despite having to work extra hard to pump blood around the increased bulk of the body. People who exercise for at least 20–30 minutes, three times per week, have a lower risk of high blood pressure, stroke, obesity and coronary heart disease than those who are physically inactive.

To be beneficial, exercise needs to be brisk enough to raise your pulse rate, produce a light sweat and to make you slightly breathless. Unfortunately, the average level of physical activity in the UK is low. Only 30 per cent of men and 20 per cent of women are active enough to gain some protection against high blood pressure. One survey among adult males found that one in five had taken no exercise at all during the preceding month. Although exercise increases the amount of blood pumped through the heart by up to 700 per cent, and puts BP up during the period of exercise itself, this is a healthy, temporary response.

Taking regular exercise helps to prevent high blood pressure by:

* burning off stress hormones that trigger arterial spasm in small blood vessels
* dilating peripheral veins
* increasing the efficiency of your cardiovascular system so your pulse rate falls
* boosting the muscle pump action of your skeletal muscles
* lowering blood fat levels
* reducing the risk of atherosclerosis.

For more information, see Chapter 21.

STRESS

High blood pressure is thought to be linked with excessive levels of stress in some people. Susceptible individuals have an overactive part of the nervous system (sympathetic nervous system) which is unusually responsive to stressful stimuli that would normally be associated with only a mild, temporary rise in blood pressure. This overactivity of sympathetic nerves probably runs in families, with stress acting as the environmental factor that triggers off the process.

In people sensitive to stress, a condition known as Gaisbock's syndrome can occur. This is a form of labile hypertension in which blood pressure levels can vary considerably. Sometimes they are high; sometimes they are low or normal. This can lead to more permanent hypertension if their lifestyle doesn't slow down. One of the most common signs of this is so-called *White Coat Hypertension* – blood pressure that shoots up on being measured in the surgery or hospital (usually by someone wearing a white coat or uniform). This can increase systolic BP by as much as 100 mmHg, although this is extreme. More commonly, white coat hypertension increases systolic BP by 20–30 mmHg. This form of hypertension is confirmed by attaching the sufferer to a 24-hour BP monitoring tape and showing that BP rises in stressful conditions, including having BP measured by a doctor, then falls again in between.

Until recently, white coat hypertension was thought to be relatively harmless. However, latest research suggests that people with this condition have just as many abnormalities of the heart and blood vessels (e.g. poor left ventricular function, decreased elasticity and increased stiffness of artery walls) as those with persistently high blood pressure. They are also likely to develop hypertension in the future.

In most people, however, stress only causes only a transient rise in BP as a result of the hormone adrenaline (epinephrine). This triggers the constriction of arteries and veins which temporarily puts blood pressure up. This is an adaptive response to help you fight or flee in dangerous situations. Blood pressure can still fall when you are at rest or asleep, however, and relaxation training is usually helpful in offsetting the effects of excessive stress.

For more information, see Chapter 21.

KELOIDS

Interestingly, people who develop an excessive scar tissue reaction to a skin wound and produce a large, lumpy, keloid scar seem to be twice as likely to develop high blood pressure as people who produce normal amounts of scar tissue. This is thought to be due to a blood protein, angiotensin II, which helps to regulate blood pressure. It is now also known to stimulate production of collagen – a fibrous protein found in scar tissue. A group of drugs that block angiotensin (angiotensin converting enzyme – or ACE-inhibitors) are commonly used to treat high blood pressure. The link is the result of much research in an attempt to unravel some of the mysteries of essential hypertension.

For more information on dietary factors affecting essential hypertension, such as increased salt intake, and low intakes of calcium, magnesium, folic acid and antioxidants, see Chapters 6, 7, and 12.

Causes of Secondary Hypertension

One in ten people with hypertension have a recognizsed, underlying cause and are said to have *secondary hypertension*. Secondary hypertension should always be ruled out in any hypertensive person, but it is especially important to exclude other conditions in people developing high blood pressure before the age of 35.

KIDNEY DISEASE

The commonest cause of secondary hypertension is kidney disease, which accounts for 8 out of 10 cases. High blood pressure can also be the cause of kidney disease, however, and it can be difficult for doctors to tell which condition developed first. When high blood pressure is the cause of kidney disease, this occurs because essential hypertension leads to hardening and furring up of the large renal arteries and also damages small blood vessels in the kidney. As a result, blood supply to the kidneys is reduced and they may start to shrink. At the same time, poor blood supply to the kidney filtering units (nephrons) means less urine is produced. Kidney function progressively deteriorates and fluid builds up in the circulation, contributing to hypertension. Poor blood supply to the kidneys also stimulates the special pressure receptors (baroreceptors) in the kidneys that are responsible for monitoring blood pressure. If they detect blood pressure has fallen within the kidneys, they trigger increased production of renin hormone, which raises blood pressure in an attempt to increase blood supply to the kidneys. This puts BP up even more, so another vicious cycle develops.

Where kidney disease comes first, and high blood pressure develops as a consequence, the usual kidney diseases involved are:

* chronic glomerulonephritis (inflammation of the kidney filtration units)
* chronic atrophic pyelonephritis (shrinking of kidney tissue due to chronic infection or inflammation)

✿ congenital polycystic kidneys (abnormal kidney structure due to the formation of multiple cysts during embryonic development).

Kidney problems are thought to cause high blood pressure by reducing filtration of excess fluid and salts from the body, which build up in the circulation to raise blood pressure. Increased secretion of renin hormone is also involved.

OTHER CAUSES

Other relatively common causes of secondary hypertension include:

✿ pre-eclampsia during the last three months of pregnancy (which affects around one in ten pregnant women)
✿ the side-effects of some drugs.

Rarer causes of secondary hypertension include:

✿ anatomical abnormalities of the circulatory system such as narrowing of the aorta or renal artery
✿ polycythaemia, in which blood stickiness is significantly increased due to over-production of red blood cells
✿ Conn's syndrome, in which there are high levels of aldosterone hormone
✿ phaeochromocytoma, due to a tumour that secretes excessive amounts of adrenaline hormone and noradrenaline
✿ Cushing's syndrome, due to excessive exposure to corticosteroids – either from overactive adrenal glands or from steroid drug treatment
✿ acromegaly, due to excessive production of growth hormone by the pituitary gland
✿ hyperparathyroidism, due to overactivity of the four parathyroid glands in the neck which, if not treated, raises blood calcium levels and can damage the kidneys.

SECONDARY HYPERTENSION DUE TO DRUGS

Several drugs – both those available on prescription and those bought over the counter – can put your blood pressure up while they are being taken. These include:

✿ nasal decongestants (e.g. ephedrine), taken to relieve a blocked nose
✿ non-steroidal anti-inflammatory drugs (e.g. ibuprofen), taken to relieve aches and pains in the muscles and joints which – can raise BP by 5 –10 mm Hg
✿ oral corticosteroids, taken for severe inflammatory conditions such as asthma or rheumatoid arthritis
✿ the combined oral contraceptive pill (containing both oestrogen and progestogen hormones), which can raise BP after several years' use – recent research suggests that the average increase in BP is around 2.8/1.9 mmHg. In some women, however, rapid and more severe rises in BP can occur
✿ monoamine-oxidase inhibitors – drugs sometimes used to treat severe depression – can cause sudden rises in BP if you eat cheese or other foods containing tyramine while on medication
✿ carbenoxolone – a synthetic version of liquorice, sometimes used to treat stomach ulcers – can

put BP up as it can trigger retention of sodium and water; a similar effect can also occur if you eat too much liquorice which has not been deglycerrizhinated.

Diagnosing High Blood Pressure

ROUTINE EXAMINATIONS

If your doctor finds your blood pressure is raised, you will probably have the following examinations:

* checking your blood pressure at least twice during the first visit
* feeling your pulse to see how regular and strong it is
* checking pulses in your groin, feet and ankles to make sure your peripheral circulation is intact – pressing on the skin of your lower legs and then letting go will show how quickly blood flows back into the blanched area
* feeling your chest to see where the tip of your beating heart is detectable – this gives a good indication of whether or not your heart is enlarged
* listening to your heart with a stethoscope to check for heart murmurs and to listen to your heart beat rhythm
* listening to your lungs to check for signs of fluid build-up on the chest
* listening to your neck and abdomen with a stethoscope to detect any noises due to turbulent blood flow through damaged carotid or renal arteries
* examining the backs of your eyes to look for any signs of arterial damage (*see below*).

If your blood pressure remains consistently raised, you may have the following routine investigations:

* chest x-ray – to check the size and shape of the heart and to look for evidence of congestive heart failure with fluid build-up on the lungs
* ECG – heart tracing to look for signs of left-ventricular thickening, irregular heartbeat or evidence that the heart muscle is struggling
* analysis of a urine sample – to look for protein and sugar, which would suggest blood vessels in the kidney are damaged
* blood test for urea and electrolytes – to check kidney function and your salt balance
* blood test for fasting blood lipids – to see if your blood cholesterol or other fat levels are raised.

If your doctor suspects your blood pressure is due to an underlying cause, you may have one or more of the following tests carried out:

* If your potassium level is low, and you are not on diuretic treatment, you may have a hormone problem leading to high blood pressure. You will therefore have blood tests taken to check levels of other hormones such as aldosterone, cortisol and renin.
* Blood tests to assess kidney function (creatinine clearance rate).
* An intravenous urogram – a substance that shows up on x-ray is injected into your blood stream

and a series of x-rays taken. This shows any narrowing of your renal arteries, how well your kidneys concentrate the dye in the urine, and outlines your urinary system to show up anatomical abnormalities or shrinkage of the kidneys.

* Ultrasound of your kidneys.
* Blood tests to measure catecholamine levels or measurement of urinary vanillylmandelic acid if phaeochromocytoma (tumour of the adrenal gland) is suspected.
* If acromegaly is suspected from changes to your facial features and the fact that your tongue, jaw, hands and feet are getting bigger, you will have your blood levels of growth hormone measured.

EYE EXAMINATIONS

High blood pressure damages small arteries throughout your body. Those in the back of the eye have the advantage of being visible using an ophthalmoscope and they show the state of arterioles throughout your system, including your brain. Early changes due to hypertension include thickening of retinal blood vessel walls. If hypertension becomes long-standing or severe, the blood vessels leak and little haemorrhages form. Other changes are probably due to obstruction of vessels and reduced blood circulation.

Your doctor will regularly check the back of your eyes for signs of damage if your blood pressure has been high. This is performed in a darkened room using an ophthalmoscope, which contains a number of lenses and a light source. Sometimes you may have one eye dilated first with drops to make the task easier. The doctor is looking for various abnormalities known as Keith-Wagener retinal changes. These are divided into four stages of severity:

* Grade 1 – retinal arteries are more tortuous i.e. less straight. Because they are thickened and bulging under pressure, they also reflect light from the ophthalmoscope more than usual. This gives them an appearance known as silver wiring.
* Grade 2 – as in grade 1, plus evidence that the thickened, bulging arteries are compressing the veins where they cross over them (arterio-venous nipping).
* Grade 3 – as in grade 2, plus signs that the arteries have started leaking. Leakage of protein-rich fluid produces white, soft, 'cotton wool'-like blobs while leakage of blood produces flame-shaped haemorrhages.
* Grade 4 – as in grade 3, plus swelling, bulging and blurring of the head of the optic nerve (papilloedema).

If haemorrhages, exudates or papilloedema are visible in the back of the eye, it shows that *malignant hypertension* (*see page 5*) has developed. These are the same sort of processes that are occurring in the brain and which are thought to lead to a stroke. It is very important that your hypertension is brought under control quickly and safely. You may be admitted to hospital for complete bed rest while your drug treatment is adjusted.

Peripheral Vascular Disease

Hardening and furring up of the arteries throughout the body can lead to peripheral vascular disease in which blood supply to your legs is severely limited. Even a mild increase in exercise means that your muscles need extra blood and oxygen – if these cannot be supplied, your leg muscles will start to cramp. This causes a severe pain in the calf muscles which comes on during exercise and stops when you rest – a condition called *intermittent claudication*. If your blood supply is severely affected, even walking 100 metres or less on the flat can bring symptoms on. If blood supply is very poor, ischaemic pain may occur at rest, tissues may break down to form a leg ulcer and eventually gangrene may set in. Severe peripheral vascular disease is most likely in someone with hypertension who also smokes, or who also suffers from diabetes.

Aspirin will help to thin the blood and improve blood supply. Some tablets also work by increasing the flexibility of red blood cells so they can squeeze through small blood vessels more easily. Interestingly, research shows that taking garlic powder tablets, ginkgo biloba or a mix of Tibetan herbs known as Padma 28 can improve peripheral circulation enough to increase the distance you can walk before calf pain starts by up to 30 per cent in three months (*see Chapter 19*).

A severely narrowed artery in the leg can be overcome with a bypass graft to open up an alternative circulatory route. If there are only one or two main sites of blockage, these can sometimes be overcome by passing a balloon catheter into the artery and expanding it at the site of blockage to locally dilate the vessel in that area.

Treatment of High Blood Pressure

Early diagnosis and treatment can control your blood pressure before it harms your health. You will have your blood pressure measured several times before your doctor will decide to prescribe any anti-hypertensive drugs. This is to make sure your blood pressure remains consistently high and is not just going up as a result of visiting the surgery. The aim of blood-pressure treatment is to reduce diastolic BP to below 85 mmHg and/or systolic BP to below 140 mmHg (thresholds may be different in some groups of people such as the very elderly). Sometimes two or even three different types of drug are needed to achieve this goal.

The aim of treatment is to lower your blood pressure gradually. Your doctor will start you off on a low dose of tablets to see how your blood pressure responds. If this is not enough, your dose may be increased, other drugs may be added in, or your medication may be completely changed. In some cases, more than one drug may be needed to achieve an acceptable BP. It may seem annoying to have to take one, two or even three different kinds of drugs when you feel perfectly well. But by prescribing treatment to keep your blood pressure within normal limits, your doctor is helping you to avoid the complications of uncontrolled hypertension – heart attack, stroke, peripheral vascular disease, kidney failure and even blindness.

It is important to take your blood pressure tablets regularly as prescribed. Some tablets only need only to be taken once a day, but others may need to be taken two or more times daily. This depends on how long each dose of medicine works in your body, and on how bad your blood pressure is.

When most forms of anti-hypertensive treatment are stopped, blood pressure only climbs up only slowly over several days or even weeks. With some forms of treatment, however, a rebound effect can occur so your blood pressure shoots back up.

Don't stop taking your blood pressure treatment without first consulting your doctor. If you notice something that may be a side-effect, such as a rash, dizziness or sexual problems, always tell your doctor immediately so your dose can be altered or your treatment changed to one that suits you better.

> Research shows that controlling hypertension can:
> - lower the risk of stroke by 35 per cent
> - reduce the risk of heart complications by 20 per cent
> - reduce overall risk of death at any age by 15 per cent.

GUIDELINES FOR DOCTORS

Doctors have been given guidelines to help them decide which patients with high blood pressure need treatment and which don't. Basically, if your BP is consistently found to be above a certain level, it is important to bring it down to normal to reduce your risk of future complications such as coronary heart disease, kidney failure, eye problems (hypertensive retinopathy) or stroke. If complications (target organ damage) are already in evidence, the management of your condition will be stepped up.

These guidelines are based on extensive studies and trials that confirm the health benefits of treatment. In some cases, where blood pressure is borderline, and research does not show clear benefits of treatment, your doctor will monitor you regularly to make sure your BP does not go up. In these cases, diet and lifestyle changes are often enough to control your BP so you don't need to take drug treatment at all.

You might find it interesting to read the guidelines given to doctors. These are as follows:

Measurement

Baseline BP is established by taking two to three BP readings per visit (while the patient is sitting) on up to four occasions.

Aims of Treatment

To reduce diastolic BP to less than 85 mmHg and to reduce systolic BP to less than 140 mmHg, but the optimal target in people with diabetes or kidney disease is lower. In the elderly, the threshold for treatment is usually higher, as research only shows consistent benefits in treating a BP that is persistently raised to 160/90 or greater.

Target Organ Damage

This is defined as left ventricle of heart enlarged; angina; transient ischaemia attacks (TIAs); stroke; peripheral vascular disease; heart attack; kidney function impaired.

- Where the initial blood pressure is systolic ≥ 220mmHg OR diastolic ≥ 120mmHg, treat immediately.
- Where the initial blood pressure is systolic 200–219 mmHg OR diastolic 110–119 mmHg, confirm over one to two weeks then treat if these values are sustained.
- Where the initial blood pressure is systolic 160–199 mmHg OR diastolic 100–109 mmHg, AND the patient has cardiovascular complications, end organ damage or diabetes (type I or II), confirm over three to four weeks then treat if these values are sustained.
- Where the initial blood pressure is systolic 160–199 mmHg OR diastolic 100–109 mmHg, but the

patient has NO cardiovascular complications, end organ damage or diabetes, advise lifestyle changes, reassess weekly initially and treat if these values are sustained on repeat measurements over four to twelve weeks.

* Where the initial blood pressure is systolic 140–159 mmHg OR diastolic 90–99 mmHg, AND the patient has cardiovascular complications, end organ damage or diabetes, confirm within four to twelve weeks and treat if these values are sustained.

* Where the initial blood pressure is systolic 140–159 mmHg OR diastolic 90–99 mmHg, but the patient has NO cardiovascular complications, end organ damage or diabetes, advise lifestyle changes, reassess monthly; if mild hypertension persists, treat if the risk of coronary heart disease is greater than or equal to 15 per cent over the next 10 years using the Joint British Societies Coronary Risk Prediction Charts (which give a predicted future CHD risk depending on age, gender, smoking status, systolic blood pressure, cholesterol levels and diabetic status).

DRUGS USED TO TREAT HYPERTENSION

At present, six classes of drug are available to lower high blood pressure:

* thiazide diuretics
* beta-blockers
* alpha-blockers
* calcium channel blockers
* ACE inhibitors
* angiotensin-II receptor antagonists.

If a single drug is not effective, other anti-hypertensive drugs may be added, usually at intervals of at least four weeks, until good control of BP is achieved. Where hypertension is relatively mild (systolic BP less than 160mmHg, and diastolic less than 100mmHg), drugs may be substituted rather than used together.

Thiazide Diuretics

Thiazide diuretics (e.g. bendrofluazide, hydrochlorothiazide) are generally used as a first-line treatment in the elderly, or are combined with other anti-hypertensive drugs (e.g. a beta-blocker or ACE inhibitor) to boost their action in younger patients.

They lower blood pressure by increasing loss of salts through the kidneys into the urine. This tends to draw fluid out of the circulation, causes mild dilation of small arteries and lowers arteriolar resistance. The diuretics act within an hour or two of being given and are usually taken in the morning so you do not have to get up at night to pass water. When you first start taking the tablets, you may notice that you have to pass water more frequently than usual for the first few days;, then this effect tends to disappear as dilation of the arterioles occurs. Only low doses of hiazide diuretic are needed to bring your diastolic BP down by around 5 mmHg – higher doses have no further effect on BP and are more likely to cause side effects such as salt imbalances.

They should not be used by people with diabetes or with sodium, potassium or calcium imbalances, severe kidney or liver problems, active gout or Addison's disease.

Beta-blockers

The way beta-blockers lower blood pressure is not fully understood but is thought to result from a combination of actions in which they:

* alter the way nerve signals cause some blood vessels to dilate or constrict
* slow the heart rate to around 60 beats per minute
* reduce the force of contraction of the heart
* decrease the workload of the heart and cardiac output
* lower secretion of a kidney hormone, renin
* reduce sensitivity of blood pressure sensors (baroreceptors)
* block stress hormone (adrenaline) receptors
* have some effects on the brain.

In general, beta-blockers are used as a first-line treatment in young people with hypertension and in people who have coronary heart disease. Because they also affect receptors in the lungs, they should not be used in people with asthma as they may trigger an asthma attack. Beta-blockers have been shown to significantly reduce the risk of having a second heart attack and may prolong life in high-risk individuals.

Beta-blockers should not be withdrawn suddenly, but must be tailed off slowly so that rebound high blood pressure (or angina) does not occur.

Alpha-blockers

Alpha-blockers (e.g. doxazosin, indoramin, prazosin, terazosin) lower blood pressure by dilating both arteries and veins. They are particularly helpful for older males who have both high blood pressure and problems associated with benign enlargement of the prostate gland. They sometimes cause a rapid fall in blood pressure after the first dose so treatment should be started with caution – usually at night so that if low blood pressure does occur, this is after you have retired to bed.

If taking Indoramin, you should avoid alcohol as it boosts alcohol absorption.

Calcium Channel Blockers

Calcium channel blockers (e.g. diltiazem, felodipine, isradipine, lacidipine, nicardipine, nifedipine) work by:

* blocking the transport of calcium ions through cell membranes
* relaxing muscles in arterial walls and reducing arterial spasm
* dilating peripheral veins to encourage pooling of blood
* dilating peripheral veins to encourage pooling of blood
* reducing the force of contraction of the heart.

Treatment must not be stopped suddenly, but should be tailed off slowly to prevent rebound angina. Verapamil is slightly different from the others in the way it works, and should not be used together with a beta-blocker.

ACE Inhibitors

ACE inhibitor drugs are so-named because they block formation of Angiotensin Converting Enzyme (ACE). This in turn prevents formation of a substance called angiotensin II – a powerful constrictor of blood vessels – leading to dilation of both small arteries and veins. This reduces total peripheral resistance and arterial blood pressure. ACE inhibitors also increase blood flow to the kidneys, so more fluid and sodium is lost as urine. They are usually considered for treating hypertension when thiazides diuretics or beta-blockers are contraindicated, not tolerated, or fail to control high blood pressure.

They can cause a sudden fall in BP on giving the first dose, especially in people who are taking diuretics or who are dehydrated. Where possible, diuretic treatment is therefore usually stopped a few days before ACE inhibitor treatment is started. For some, the first dose is best taken at night on retiring to bed. Kidney function and salt balance should be checked before treatment is started. ACE inhibitors may be less effective in people of Afro-Caribbean descent unless combined with a thiazide diuretic.

Angiotensin- II Receptor Antagonists

These drugs (e.g. losartan, valsartan, candesartan) are similar to the ACE inhibitors except that instead of inhibiting angiotensin-converting enzyme, they block angiotensin-II to produce similar effects. This dilates blood vessels, stimulates kidney function and may also have a direct action on the brain to reduce drinking and increase urine output. At present, they are mainly used in people who develop a persistent dry cough as a troublesome side-effect of the ACE inhibitors as these particular drugs do not produce this problem.

Other Drugs

Occasionally, drugs from the above groups may not be sufficient or suitable for treating an individual case of high blood pressure. Two other drugs are sometimes used: hydralazine or methyldopa.

Hydralazine is a vasodilator that lowers blood pressure by relaxing arteries and increasing their diameter. When used to treat hypertension, it is usually combined with a beta-blocker and thiazide diuretic to stop the heart rate and cardiac output from increasing and to avoid fluid retention. It may cause a very rapid drop in blood pressure.

Methyldopa used to be the most popular drug for treating high blood pressure, and may still be taken by elderly patients who started on it many years ago. It lowers blood pressure by acting on the brain to trigger nerve actions that reduce heart output, urine production and arteriolar constriction. Methyldopa is often used together with a diuretic. It may cause a rapid fall in blood pressure, especially in the elderly.

Your doctor may also suggest taking low-dose aspirin or taking drugs to lower blood cholesterol levels if necessary.

IS ANTI-HYPERTENSIVE TREATMENT FOR LIFE?

Once drug treatment is started for high blood pressure, it is often for life. However, if you don't have any complications from your high blood pressure and you have managed to make diet and lifestyle changes that naturally bring your blood pressure down, it may be possible to reduce your tablet dose or to withdraw it altogether. However, you should never alter your medication or stop it suddenly yourself. If your doctor decides to withdraw your treatment, this is usually done slowly in a step-wise fashion to prevent a sudden rebound hypertension. You will be followed up closely over a long period of time, as, in some cases, BP starts to creep back up again after six months, a year or more.

IF YOU SHOULD FORGET TO TAKE YOUR MEDICATION

If you do forget to take your treatment occasionally, it is unlikely that you will come to any harm. If you forget your tablets on a regular basis, however, you may run into problems.

* If your treatment is only a few hours late, take it as soon as you remember.
* If you have missed one dose and your next one is already due, just take one dose – DON'T take an extra dose next time. Be especially careful not to miss any further doses.
* If you forget to take your blood blood-pressure treatment for more than one or two days, contact your doctor for further advice.

Tips to Help You Remember to Take Your Medication

* Try to take your blood-pressure treatment regularly, at the same time every day, so you get into a routine.
* Write a note for yourself and stick it where you will easily see it.
* Keep your tablets/capsules where you can remember them easily, such as with your toothpaste (but make sure they are out of the reach of children).
* Keep your tablets in a special dispenser box marked with separate containers for different times of the day.
* If you have a programmable alarm watch, set it for when your medicine is due.
* If you live with someone else, ask them to help you remember .
* Make sure you get your next prescription in plenty of time so you don't run out.
* If you are going away, take enough tablets with you to last the whole time.

DRUGS TO LOWER HIGH BLOOD CHOLESTEROL

The best way to reduce high cholesterol is through making dietary changes and increasing the amount of exercise you take. Doctors usually recommend a low- fat diet, using olive or rapeseed oil for cooking, eating oily fish, taking fish oil supplements and garlic powder tablets.

If dietary changes have failed, your doctor may prescribe a lipid-lowering drug. This would be in instances where total blood cholesterol is above 7.8 mmol/l and is mainly in the form of harmful LDL-cholesterol.

In some cases, raised cholesterol levels are due to hereditary difficulties with fat metabolism. In these instances, one or more drugs often have to be prescribed.

Resins

Resins (e.g. cholestyramine, colestipol) work by binding to bile acids and preventing their re-absorption in the gut. This interferes with regulatory messages feeding back to the liver, so that more cholesterol is broken down into bile acids and excreted from the body. These drugs can lower LDL-cholesterol levels by up to 25 per cent on top of that achieved through dietary changes. Unfortunately, they cause triglycerides – another type of dietary fat linked to heart disease – to rise by up to 5 per cent. They are mainly used when a statin cannot be taken (*see below*). Side-effects include constipation and, in long-term treatment, a lack of fat-soluble vitamins A, D, E and K.

Fibrates

Fibrates (e.g. bezafibrate, ciprofibrate, clofibrate, fenofibrate, gemfibrozil) work by lowering liver synthesis of cholesterol. They reduce total cholesterol by up to 25 per cent and triglycerides by up to 50 per cent. They also have a beneficial effect on types of cholesterol in the blood, raising HDL and lowering LDL cholesterol. Unfortunately, they can trigger muscle pain (myositis), especially in patients with kidney disease. Some encourage gallstones and inflammation of the gall bladder by increasing excretion of cholesterol into the bile. Other possible side-effects include fatigue, muscle cramps, dizziness, painful extremities, hair loss, blurred vision, impotence and, rarely, inability to feel sexual pleasure.

Statins

Statins (e.g. fluvastatin, pravastatin, simvastatin) work by inhibiting a liver enzyme and lowering cholesterol production in the liver. LDL-cholesterol can be reduced by up to 40 per cent, with a beneficial rise in HDL-cholesterol and a moderate reduction in triglycerides. Statins are very pop-ular drugs as they significantly reduce the risk of heart disease and stroke. Side-effects include reversible muscle problems, non-cardiac chest pain, diarrhoea, constipation, sinusitis, insomnia, flatulence and fatigue. Side-effects may be reduced by taking co-enzyme Q10 supplements.

Nicotinic Acid Derivatives

These drugs (e.g. acipimox, nicofuranose, nicotinic acid) lower both triglycerides and cholesterol levels by inhibiting the breakdown of body fat stores and the inhibiting production of fats in the liver. LDL-cholesterol can be lowered by up to 20 per cent and HDL-cholesterol is increased. They are limited by their side-effects of dilating the blood vessels dilation, causing dizziness, headaches and flushing.

Marine Fish Oils

Marine omega-3-triglycerides are a natural product that reduces blood levels of cholesterol and harmful triglycerides by inhibiting their production in the liver. They make the blood less sticky and reduce the risk of arterial thrombosis. They have few side-effects apart from possible nausea (if too much is taken) and belching. If diabetic, monitor blood gluscose levels carefully when starting to take them.

Probucal

This drug is in a class of its own, and its precise mode of action is unknown. It seems to increase excretion of bile acids in the faeces, so that more cholesterol is broken down in the liver to replenish them. It can lower LDL-cholesterol by up to 10 per cent, but HDL-cholesterol is reduced as well.

Triglycerides remain unchanged. Probucal also acts as an antioxidant. Possible side-effects include flatulence, diarrhoea, mild abdominal pain and, very rarely, abnormal heart rhythm.

Aspirin

Aspirin is a commonly used pain killer and anti-inflammatory drug that also has a powerful blood-thinning effect. It lowers the stickiness of platelet particles in the blood so that they are less likely to clump together and form unwanted clots. This effect occurs at only a quarter of the dose needed to relieve pain. Although there is not yet felt to be enough evidence to recommend that everyone takes preventive aspirin, people who may be advised to take a regular mini-dose of aspirin every day include those who have:

* angina
* had a heart attack
* had a coronary artery by-pass graft or dilation (angioplasty)
* had surgery for poor circulation in the limbs
* diabetes
* several major risk factors for CHD.

Studies show that taking low-dose aspirin (75mg–150 mg) per day can reduce the risk of a heart attack or stroke by 30 per cent, and the risk of dying from them by 15 per cent (*see Chapter 3*).

If you fall into any of the above groups and are not taking a junior aspirin per day, check with your doctor that it will suit you and fit in with any other medication that you are taking.

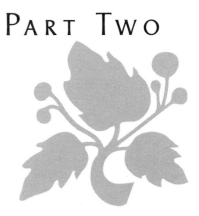

PART TWO

High Blood Pressure and Diet

CHAPTER 3

Atherosclerosis, Cholesterol and Dietary Fats

People with hypertension need to pay particular attention to the fats in their diet. By eating more of certain beneficial fats and less of potentially harmful ones, you can reduce your risk of future complications such as atherosclerosis.

Atherosclerosis

Atherosclerosis is the medical term for hardening, furring up and narrowing of the arteries. This process starts early in life, usually in the teens, and is triggered by normal wear-and-tear damage to your artery walls. Once the damage occurs, small cell fragments in the bloodstream – known as platelets – stick to the damaged area and form a tiny clot. These platelets release chemical signals to stimulate healing of the damaged area. Under normal circumstances, this would lead to healing, but if excessive damage continues – as a result of high blood pressure, raised cholesterol levels, poorly controlled diabetes or lack of antioxidants in the diet – the damaged area becomes infiltrated with a porridge-like substance that builds up to form a fatty plaque known as atheroma.

At the same time as the fatty plaques are developing, the underlying middle layer of the artery wall is affected and starts to degenerate, become fibrous and less compliant. Whereas the walls of healthy arteries are elastic and help to even out the surges of blood pressure produced every time the heart beats, the walls of arteries that have started to harden become more rigid. As a result, blood-pressure surges caused by the heartbeat are not evened out, and systolic blood pressure shoots up higher when the heart contracts. A vicious cycle then sets up, for just as atherosclerosis leads to high blood pressure, untreated hypertension can also lead to atherosclerosis by damaging artery linings and hastening the hardening and furring-up process.

If atherosclerosis is widespread throughout the body, it narrows the circulation so the diastolic BP – the pressure in the system when the heart is resting between beats – also becomes raised. Atherosclerosis can therefore raise both diastolic and systolic blood pressure. If left untreated, the raised BP in turn causes damage to the arterial system, hastening the development of atherosclerotic plaques and causing blood pressure to rise even further.

As a result, the heart has to pump blood out into a circulation whose vessels are narrowed and have lost their elasticity. This increases the workload of the heart – which has to pump blood out into the high-pressure system – and its need for oxygen increases at a time when its blood supply is often already compromised due to atherosclerosis of the coronary arteries. As the heart muscle beats over 100,000 times per day, lack of oxygen rapidly leads to muscle cramping, making angina and a heart attack more likely. In some people, two-thirds or more of a coronary artery may be furred up and blocked without causing symptoms. In others, angina may be triggered even though only a small plaque is present and the coronary artery is narrowed only slightly. It all depends on:

* the exact site where the atheroma and narrowing have developed – the most common is within 3cm of where a coronary artery originates from the aorta, so the effects of ischaemia (lack of blood supply) are likely to be more widespread and serious
* how well the two main coronary arteries join up to share the load of supplying blood
* how good the blood supply from the other coronary artery is
* the type of coronary arteries you have inherited – whether they are the vascular equivalent of motorways or winding country lanes.

Cholesterol Levels

Fats from your food are processed in the small intestines to form fatty globules (chylomicrons) bound to carrier proteins, which together form substances known as lipoproteins. After a fatty meal, there may be so many of these fatty particles in the circulation that blood takes on a milky-white appearance. These fatty globules are cleared from your bloodstream by the action of an enzyme (lipoprotein lipase) found in the walls of blood capillaries. Some of the fat released in this way is taken up into cells, while some remains in the circulation and is transported to the liver. In the liver, the fats are processed, packaged to different types of carrier proteins and passed out into the circulation again for further distribution around your body.

There are two main types of circulating cholesterol:

* low-density lipoprotein (LDL) cholesterol, which is linked with hardening and furring up of artery walls, high blood pressure and coronary heart disease
* high-density lipoprotein (HDL) cholesterol, which protects against atherosclerosis and CHD by transporting LDL-cholesterol away from the arteries for metabolism.

Research shows that for every 1 per cent rise in beneficial HDL cholesterol, there is a corresponding fall in the risk of CHD of as much as 2 per cent. This seems to be due to reversed cholesterol transport in which HDL moves LDL cholesterol away from the tissues and back towards the liver.

It is, therefore, not so much your total blood cholesterol level that is important when it comes to atherosclerosis but the ratio between beneficial HDL cholesterol and harmful LDL cholesterol. If you are told you have a raised blood cholesterol level, it is important to know whether your LDL or HDL cholesterol is high:

* if your blood fats consist mainly of HDL-cholesterol, your risk of CHD is significantly reduced
* if most of the lipids are in the form of LDL-cholesterol, with low HDL levels, your risk of CHD is

significantly increased. Ideally, total cholesterol level should be less than 5mmol/l, with LDL cholesterol less than 3mmol/l.

Where LDL cholesterol levels are raised, it is estimated that reducing the average total blood cholesterol level by 10 per cent could prevent over a quarter of all deaths due to coronary heart disease. Unfortunately, attempts to reduce dietary cholesterol for improved cardiovascular health often have the opposite effect. Rather than just lowering the potentially harmful LDL form of cholesterol, dietary interventions often reduce levels of beneficial HDL-cholesterol as well. This is because the types of fat in your diet are also important, and people often cut out the good fats as well as the less desirable ones. If you ate all your fat in the form of essential fatty acids, mono-unsaturated fats (e.g. olive oil) and fish oils, for example, your risk of CHD would be low as most circulating fats would be in the form of beneficial HDL-cholesterol.

Dietary Fats, Atherosclerosis and Inflammation

Research into atherosclerosis has suggested that dietary fats play an important role in its development. Atherosclerosis is now known to be a chronic inflammatory process as it involves certain blood cells, known as monocytes, that only leave the circulation and enter body tissues if inflammation is present. Once monocytes leave the blood, they become known as macrophages and act as scavenger cells, which are attracted to foreign substances to help mop them up. The fatty plaques that develop in damaged arterial walls are full of these scavenger cells that have become so overburdened with globules of fat that they die and accumulate in artery walls.

The most popular theory is that macrophages mistake certain fats in the diet for invading bacteria. The monocytes leave the bloodstream and enter the artery wall in an attempt to engulf these 'foreign' fats and destroy them. They aim a cocktail of powerful chemicals against the fat to oxidize it, setting up an inflammatory reaction that attracts more macrophages into the area. The most harmful molecules come from oxidation of a type of fat called omega-6 polyunsaturated fatty acid.

WHY YOU NEED FATS

Ideally, dietary fats should provide between 25 and 30 per cent of daily energy, although dietary guidelines in the UK currently give 35 per cent as the upper limit. Unfortunately, food surveys suggest that, for the average adult, dietary fats currently provide over 40 per cent of daily calories, which is far too high. Most people would benefit from cutting back on their overall fat intake while increasing their intake of the more beneficial types of fat.

A certain amount of fat is important for health, as it supplies:

* energy
* essential fatty acids (linoleic acid, linolenic acid) that cannot be synthesized from other dietary fats in the body
* building blocks for cell membranes
* fatty acids necessary for the central nervous system

- precursors for making hormones and hormone-like chemicals called prostaglandins
- molecules from which bile salts are made
- fat-soluble vitamins A, D, E and K.

Eating too much saturated fat has been blamed for weight gain and – until recently – was thought to be the main culprit in raising blood cholesterol levels and triggering atherosclerosis. Researchers now increasingly believe that it is eating too much omega-6 polyunsaturated fatty acids (found mainly in vegetable oils) and not enough omega-3 polyunsaturated fatty acids (found mainly in fish oils) that increases your risk of atherosclerosis and other inflammatory diseases such as eczema, asthma, inflammatory bowel disorders and arthritis. This is especially true if your intake of antioxidants (such as vitamins C and E, betacarotene and the mineral selenium) is low. Antioxidants, which are found mainly in fresh fruit and vegetables, help to protect body fats from a chemical alteration known as oxidation (*see Chapter 19*).

TYPES OF DIETARY FAT

The fats in your diet consist of a molecule of glycerol to which three fatty-acid chains are attached sideways on to form a molecular shape similar to a capital E. The length of the fatty-acid chains, and whether or not any of their carbon atoms are linked by a double bond, dictate whether the fat is solid or liquid at room temperature, and how it is metabolized in your body.

Fats that contain no double bonds are referred to as saturated fats. Fats containing some double bonds are known as unsaturated fats – those with one double bond are monounsaturated, while those with two or more double bonds are polyunsaturated.

Most dietary fats contain a blend of saturates, monounsaturates and polyunsaturates in varying proportions. In general, saturated fats tend to be solid at room temperature while monounsaturated and polyunsaturated fats tend to be liquid, such as oils.

Polyunsaturated Fats

Unlike saturated fats, polyunsaturated fatty acids (PUFAs) have a molecular structure containing spare double bonds. This makes them highly reactive and more susceptible to chemical change through free-radical attack (such as when attacked by chemicals released by macrophages). This chemical change – known as oxidation – produces toxic substances (lipid peroxides) that are believed to trigger hardening and furring up of artery walls. Factors that encourage the formation of toxic lipid peroxides include:

- eating excessive amounts of PUFAs
- lack of dietary antioxidants
- overheating of PUFA oils so they smoke while cooking
- reusing oils over and over again.

There are two main types of polyunsaturated fat in the diet:

- omega-3 PUFAs, derived mainly from fish oils
- omega-6 PUFAs, derived mainly from vegetable oils.

Your body handles omega-3 and omega-6 oils in different ways. Omega-3 fish oils have a thinning effect on your blood and help to reduce the risk of coronary heart disease and stroke; while omega-6 PUFAs are increasingly thought to be linked with inflammatory processes in the body. Many researchers now believe the rise in numbers of people with inflammatory diseases such as CHD, asthma, rheumatoid arthritis and inflammatory bowel conditions is due to low dietary intakes of omega-3 PUFAs and increased intakes of omega-6s. The average Western diet currently contains a ratio of omega-6 to omega-3 fats of around 7:1, which is far too high.

Ideally, polyunsaturated fats should supply between 6 per cent and 10 per cent of energy intake.

Trans-Fatty Acids

When polyunsaturated oils are partially hydrogenated to solidify them in the production of cooking fats and spreads, such as margarine, some trans-fatty acids are produced. When trans-fatty acids are incorporated into your cell membranes, they increase their rigidity and also seem to raise blood levels of harmful LDL-cholesterol while lowering beneficial HDL-cholesterol. Trans-fatty acids have therefore been linked with an increased risk of high blood pressure and coronary heart disease. They may also interfere with the way your body handles essential fatty acids so their beneficial effects are not fully realized.

The average consumption of dietary trans-fatty acids is around 5–7g per day. Some people eat as much as 25–30g of trans-fatty acids per day, particularly if they use cheap margarines and lots of processed foods. Concern about their safety is such that some margarines and low-fat spreads are being reformulated to reduce their trans-fat content. Some countries have also introduced guidelines aimed at reducing intakes of trans-fatty acids from margarine from 5g per day to no more than 2g per day. In the UK, it is recommended that trans-fatty acids should supply no more than 2 per cent of your total energy intake.

Trans-fatty acids are also produced in the rumen of cattle, sheep and goats. Small amounts of trans-fats (2–4 per cent) are therefore found in milk, cheese, butter and meat. These naturally occurring trans-fats are structurally different from those produced commercially during hydrogenation of fats, however, and have not been implicated in increasing the risk of coronary heart disease.

All this has turned the butter versus margarine controversy on its head. Some scientists now believe it is healthier to eat butter rather than margarine or low-fat spreads. The simplest advice is to eat as wide a variety of foods as possible, including a little of everything (such as butter and margarine) and to eat nothing to excess.

Essential Fatty Acids

The essential fatty acids (EFAs) cannot be synthesized in your body from other dietary fats and must therefore come from your food. There are two EFAs:

- linoleic acid – an omega-6 PUFA
- linolenic acid – an omega-3 PUFA.

A third fatty acid, arachidonic acid – an omega-6 PUFA – may be essential if supplies of other EFAs (from which it can be made in the body) are low.

Unfortunately, as many as eight out of ten people do not get enough EFAs from their diet. In addition, the metabolic pathways through which your body converts one EFA into another are easily blocked by lifestyle factors. These include consuming too much saturated fat, sugar or alcohol; a lack of vitamins and minerals; smoking cigarettes; and being under excessive stress.

EFAs are important because they act as building blocks for fatty structures in your body, including those found in your cell membranes and arterial walls. If your intake of EFAs is low, your body can use the next best fats available (such as saturated fats, omega-6 PUFAs and trans-fats) and incorporate them into your cell walls. This can affect the elasticity and quality of your arteries, however, so that they are more prone to damage from high blood pressure and to atherosclerosis. EFAs also act as building blocks for hormones and hormone-like chemicals called prostaglandins. Lack of EFAs has therefore been linked to a wide range of health problems from dry, itchy or inflamed skin to hormonal problems such as acne, prostate problems and low sex drive.

EFAs are found in nuts, seeds, green leafy vegetables, oily fish, wholegrains or by taking supplements such as evening primrose, flaxseed, starflower, hemp or omega-3 fish oils.

Ideally, linoleic acid should supply at least 1 per cent of your energy intake, and linolenic acid at least 0.2 per cent.

Dietary Sources of Essential Fatty Acids
- Linoleic acid alone is found in sunflower seeds, almonds, corn, sesame seeds, pumpkin seeds, safflower oil and extra virgin olive oil.
- Linolenic acid alone is found in evening primrose oil, starflower (borage) seed oil and blackcurrant seed oil.
- Both linoleic and linolenic acids are found in rich quantities in walnuts, soya beans, linseed oil, rapeseed oil and flax oil.
- Arachidonic acid is found in many foods (e.g. seafood, meat, dairy products) and can also be made from linoleic or linolenic acids.

Monounsaturated Fats

Monounsaturated fats consist of chains of carbon atoms in which there is only one double (unsaturated) bond. Monounsaturated fats are metabolized in such a way that they lower LDL-cholesterol levels with no effect on HDL levels. Ideally, they should supply around 12 per cent of your energy intake. For most people, this means eating more monounsaturates in place of omega-6 PUFAs, which would help to reduce the risk of CHD as well as bringing the dietary ratio of omega-3s and omega-6s into a better balance. A diet high in monounsaturated fats may help to reduce your risk of atherosclerosis, high blood pressure, coronary heart disease and stroke. This is thought to explain some of the benefits of the so-called Mediterranean diet. Foods rich in monounsaturates include olive oil, rapeseed oil and avocado.

Saturated Fats

Saturated (animal) fats are converted into cholesterol in the liver. These used to be thought of as the baddies when it came to coronary heart disease but are now considered less important. As some experts have pointed out, it is unlikely that saturated fats are so harmful, given that saturated fat is the form in which your body prefers to store its excess calories.

Over a third of saturated fats in milk fat or butter (those with chain lengths of up to 10 carbon atoms and in excess of 16) have no effect on blood cholesterol levels. Only saturated fats with carbon chains of 12, 14 and 16 have any reported effect. Stearic acid (18 carbon atoms), found in milk fat, cocoa butter and meat fat, has no cholesterol-raising activity.

One of the longest-running studies into CHD found no link between high blood cholesterol levels and saturated fat intake. In fact, analysis of data from the Framingham Heart Study found that, while saturated fat intake increased as a proportion of energy from 16.4 per cent (1966–69), to 17.0 per cent (1984–88), significant decreases in blood total and LDL-cholesterol levels occurred. A recent analysis of trials involving over 30,000 people also found that altering dietary fat intake reduced cardiovascular mortality by 9 per cent, yet overall deaths were only reduced by 2 per cent.

During their epic, unassisted journey across the Antarctic in 1992, Sir Ranulph Fiennes and Dr Michael Stroud ate over 5,500 calories a day, including twice as much fat as recommended – mostly in the form of butter. Regular blood tests collected throughout the journey showed their total blood cholesterol levels did not rise, and that their level of beneficial HDL-cholesterol, which protects against CHD, went up while their level of harmful LDL-cholesterol went down.

Researchers now increasingly believe that coronary heart disease (CHD) is not so much linked to abnormally raised blood-cholesterol levels, but to a lack of dietary antioxidants (such as vitamins C and E, carotenoids, selenium). This is because antioxidants help to protect circulating fats from chemical attack (oxidation) as it is only oxidized LDL-cholesterol that is attacked by circulating scavenger cells and taken into artery walls where they contribute to the hardening and furring-up process.

This does not mean, however, that a diet high in saturated fat is harmless. Like all fats, it has a high calorie content and excess intake is linked with obesity and related complications, such as high blood pressure. Also, if you have a family history of atherosclerosis, coronary heart disease or high blood cholesterol levels, you may have inherited genes that mean you process saturated fat less well than other people. Some research has even suggested that saturated fat intake may contribute to high blood pressure, although the mechanism is unclear. When a group of people cut back on saturated fats, their systolic BP dropped by an average of 7.5mmHg and diastolic by 2.8mmHg – even though their intake of sodium chloride (salt) remained the same. When they went back to their previous high-saturated-fat diet, however, their blood pressure rose to their previous higher levels.

In the UK, guidelines recommend that no more than 35 per cent of food energy intake should come from fat and no more than 10 per cent from saturated fats, although these figures are intended as population averages, not as targets for individuals. The recommended proportions of energy provided by the various types of fat are as follows:

- monounsaturated fatty acids – 12 per cent
- polyunsaturated fatty acids – 6 per cent (maximum 10 per cent)
  - linoleic acid – 1 per cent (minimum)
  - linolenic acid – 0.2 per cent (minimum)

* trans-fatty acids – 2 per cent
* saturated fatty acids – 10 per cent.

For people with high blood pressure or other cardiovascular problems, however, I would recommend obtaining a total of no more than 30 per cent of energy intake in the form of fat. This is the upper limit suggested in some other countries, such as the US.

The average woman should aim to eat no more than around 66g of fat per day, of which monounsaturated fats should ideally predominate. For men, the average fat intake should be no more than 100g per day.

Check labels for information on the amount of fat provided by different foods, and aim for those that are as low in fat as possible.

High Blood Pressure and Plant Sterols

Back in the 1950s, scientists discovered that plant sterols, found in virtually all plants, can help to reduce absorption of cholesterol from the gut. This is because they have a similar chemical structure to animal cholesterol, which allows them to compete for sterol esterase enzymes and receptors in the intestines, so less cholesterol is absorbed.

Research has found that consuming 2g of plant sterols, or related substances known as stanols, per day, can significantly lower LDL-cholesterol and help to protect against heart disease. Modern food processing methods, unfortunately, destroy a large percentage of the naturally occurring plant sterols in our diet, so on average we only obtain between 160mg and 250mg per day. Vegetarians tend to consume twice as much but we need almost 14 times this amount for a demonstrable cholesterol-lowering effect.

A number of 'functional foods' have been developed that are fortified with additional amounts of these cholesterol-lowering substances. These include spreads and yoghurts such as Benecol and Flora pro.activ. When included in a healthy diet, they help to lower LDL-cholesterol by up to 15 per cent within as little as three weeks. For example, research has found that consuming 20–25g of a spread containing plant sterols can lower LDL-cholesterol by 10–15 per cent. This beneficial effect results from their ability to halve the amount of cholesterol absorbed from the diet, even though pre-formed dietary cholesterol only accounts for around one-eighth of the cholesterol found in the circulation (seven times more cholesterol is produced in the liver from dietary saturated fats than is obtained pre-formed in the diet).

Getting a Healthy Balance of Fats

If you suffer from high blood pressure, you can help to reduce your risk of atherosclerosis, coronary heart disease and stroke by manipulating your dietary fats so that the ratio between your HDL-cholesterol and LDL-cholesterol levels increases:

* Reduce your overall consumption of fat so that it makes up no more than 30 per cent of your daily energy intake – with saturated fat ideally comprising no more than 15 per cent of daily calories.

* Eat more monounsaturated fats (such as olive or rapeseed oils).
* Increase your intake of omega-3 fatty acids (found mainly in fish oils – *see Chapter 19*).
* Include foods fortified with plant sterols/stanols in your diet.
* Reduce your intake of omega-6 fatty acids (found mainly in vegetable oils).
* Eat as few processed foods as possible to reduce your intake of trans-fatty acids and hidden fats.

How to Cut Back on Fat

The simplest way to cut back on dietary fat is to avoid obviously fatty foods (such as doughnuts, chips, crisps and chocolate) as much as possible, and to choose reduced-fat versions of foods such as dairy products, which provide other important nutrients like calcium.

* Obtain at least half your daily calories from complex carbohydrates such as wholegrain bread and pasta, brown rice, cereals and baked potatoes, but don't smother them in calorific sauces or spreads.
* Steam, boil, dry-bake or poach food rather than deep-frying.
* Grill food rather than frying to help drain fat away. Use only a light brushing of olive or rapeseed oil if necessary plus herbs, lemon juice and spices for flavour.
* When stir-frying, use a light brushing of monounsaturated fat (such as olive or rapeseed oil).
* If roasting meat, place the meat on a rack within the roasting pan so fats drain away. Roast potatoes with just a light brushing of olive oil.
* Use skimmed or semi-skimmed rather than whole-milk products.
* Use low-fat versions of as many foods as possible, such as mayonnaise, yoghurts, salad dressings, cheese, monounsaturated spreads.
* Decrease the amount of red meat you eat to only once or twice per week. Have more vegetarian meals instead, which include pulses and beans for protein.
* Trim all visible fat from meat.
* Research suggests that eating 3g or more of soluble oat fibre per day (roughly equal to two large bowls of porridge) can lower total blood cholesterol levels by up to 0.16mm/l by absorbing fats in the gut. This slows their absorption so the body can handle them more easily. This is a small, but significant change.

The drugs used to treat high cholesterol levels are discussed at the end of Chapter 2.

CHAPTER 4

High Blood Pressure and Olive Oil

Olive oil has many desirable effects in the body and forms an important component of the heart-friendly Mediterranean diet. It is derived from the fruit of the olive tree (*Olea europaea*), which is not considered fully productive until it is 50–75 years old.

All olives start off green, as unripened fruit with a firm skin and slightly bitter taste. As the olive ripens, it passes through various shades of purple to black, and the flesh becomes increasingly wrinkly. The flavour also mellows as the oil content increases.

Olives intended for producing oil are picked when unripe as these have the lowest acid content and produce better oil. Extra-virgin olive oil is the best quality and has not been purified. Only around 10 per cent of oil produced is of this premium-grade quality. It has a distinctive green hue and is often cloudy at room temperature. Its flavour is superb as it comes from the first pressing of the fruit and retains the fresh, olive aroma with less than one per cent acidity. It also has the highest antioxidant content (vitamin E, carotenoids and polyphenols).

Virgin olive oil comes next in quality, with an acidity level of not more than 1.5 per cent. Virgin olive oil is also a premium product as it is not purified and has a slightly piquant taste.

Pure olive oil is a blend of refined oils mixed with virgin oil to provide flavour and a quality suitable for cooking. Acidity must be no more than 1.5 per cent and, although the flavour is less pleasing, this is the most widely sold oil as it is less expensive. Many are processed with olive leaves to give a green colour that mimics that of first-pressing, extra-virgin olive oils.

The major problem with olive oil is that it ages rapidly. As the oil matures, extra acidity is gained, which detracts from the original flavour. Most oils are best used within one year of pressing. If left longer than this, stale or even rancid flavours can develop, so don't store olive oil alongside your clarets! All types of olive oil should ideally be kept somewhere cool and dark, and used fresh – buy from outlets where turnover is high – and avoid large containers (especially those made from tin or aluminium). It is best bought in small sizes and renewed frequently.

---

1 tablespoon olive oil contains 15g total fat, 2g saturated fat
1 tablespoon butter contains 12g total fat, 8g saturated fat

Heart Health Benefits of Olive Oil

Olive oil is one of the healthiest dietary oils as it has beneficial effects on blood lipid levels. Its principal component – oleic acid – is processed in the body to lower total blood cholesterol. Significantly, it does this by only lowering the undesirable low-density LDL-cholesterol without modifying the beneficial high-density HDL-cholesterol. This is believed to partly explain why the incidence of coronary heart disease, high blood pressure, peripheral vascular disease, stroke and other cholesterol-related illnesses – including dementia – is low in Mediterranean regions where olive oil is used liberally for culinary and medicinal purposes.

As well as lowering abnormally raised LDL-cholesterol levels, the protective effects of olive oil against cardiovascular disease, diabetes, arthritis and even some cancers – especially breast, prostate and colon – are now well accepted. These health benefits come from its antioxidants – especially vitamin E – and its principal monounsaturated fat, oleic acid, which is an omega-9 fatty acid. Oleic acid also reduces abnormal blood-clotting tendencies and has beneficial effects on insulin levels and diabetes.

A diet rich in olive oil (34 per cent total fat, with 21 per cent as monounsaturated fatty acid and only 7 per cent as saturated fat) has been shown to reduce the risk of coronary heart disease by 25 per cent. In a study involving 605 people recovering from a heart attack, those following a Mediterranean-style diet were 56 per cent less likely to have another heart attack, or to die from heart problems, than those following their normal diet.

Among people with high blood pressure, using 30–40g of olive oil for cooking every day has been shown to reduce their need for anti-hypertensive drugs by almost 50 per cent over a six-month period, compared with only 4 per cent for those using sunflower oil. All those on the sunflower oil diet continued to need their anti-hypertensive drug treatment, while 80 per cent of those using olive oil were able to discontinue their drug treatment altogether. This effect was thought to be related to the antioxidant polyphenols in olive oil.

The ideal intake appears to be at least 10g, and preferably 30–40g, daily. For those who do not cook their own food, or who have little opportunity to include extra-virgin olive oil in their diet, extra-virgin olive oil capsules are now widely available as a supplement.

Cooking with Olive Oil

According to researchers at the University of Münster in Germany, olive oil remains stable at elevated temperatures due to its high levels of monounsaturated fatty acids and natural antioxidant, vitamin E. Refined olive oil can therefore be heated up to 210 degrees Celsius before chemical changes take place. Virgin and extra-virgin olive oils are less stable, however, due to their higher content of heat-sensitive components that contribute to their colour and flavour. Because of this, virgin olive oil may cause unwanted smells or taste changes if heated above 180 degrees Celsius. Fry with pure olive oil and keep virgin or extra-virgin olive oils for steaming, braising and salad dressings. As with other oils, oxidation occurs over time. Store properly and use while fresh (*see above*). Discard any oil that begins to smoke or smell odd during use. Ideally, cooking oils should not be reused.

Olive Oil for Salad Dressing

Only use fresh extra-virgin or virgin olive oil for salad dressings. The following recipe for a herb oil is excellent for basting fish during grilling (broiling), or for drizzling over salad. It takes two weeks to mature and stores well.

Mediterranean Herb Oil

500ml (18fl oz/2[1/4] cups) extra-virgin olive oil

10 black peppercorns

10 green peppercorns

10 fennel seeds

10 coriander (cilantro) seeds

1 sprig rosemary

1 sprig thyme

1 sprig tarragon

1 sprig oregano

1 bay leaf

2 cloves garlic, peeled and scored

2 red chili peppers

1 tsp rock salt

Place all ingredients in a clear wine bottle and cork. Shake well. Leave for two weeks, in a sun-lit place if possible, before using.

CHAPTER 5

High Blood Pressure and Oily Fish

Fish features regularly in the diets of the healthiest peoples in the world – especially those with the lowest risk of coronary heart disease, such as people eating Mediterranean and Eskimo diets.

Eating oily fish two or three times a week has been shown to reduce the risk of heart attack, stroke, inflammatory bowel disease, rheumatoid arthritis and psoriasis. In fact, eating oily fish at least twice a week can lower your risk of CHD more than following a low-fat, high-fibre diet. Research also shows that the protective effects of oily fish are seen after only six months and, after two years, those on a high-fish diet are almost a third less likely to die from CHD than those not eating much fish. This rapid action is thought to result from a thinning effect on the blood, which reduces the chance of blood clots.

These beneficial effects are derived from several essential fatty acids found in fish oils that were originally derived from algae eaten throughout the fish's life. One of the most important of these for circulatory health is EPA (eicosapentanoic acid), while others such as DHA (docosahexaenoic acid) help to maintain healthy nerve cell membranes.

Fish oils have such a powerful, beneficial effect on health that some experts recommend you eat at least 300g of oily fish (such as mackerel, herring, salmon, trout, sardines, pilchards) per week. For most people, this means eating 10 times more fish than usual! Non-oily fish also contains some beneficial oils and should ideally feature in a diet that helps you beat high blood pressure.

Unfortunately, due to concerns about pollutants such as heavy metals, dioxins and chemicals known as PCBs, the UK Food Standards Agency recently suggested eating oily fish only once a week. If you want to eat more, try to obtain fish classed as organic, or consider taking fish oil supplements that have been checked for safe levels of pollutants.

Selecting Really Fresh Fish

Never be afraid to ask your fishmonger if you can inspect the fish. After all, you're the one who has to eat it – and suffer in the bathroom if it's off.

Fresh fish should smell of seawater – salty, with a tang of ozone and slightly sweet. It should not smell of fish. This characteristic smell comes from the breakdown of chemicals, so if your fish smells fishy, it's a sure sign it's not as fresh as possible.

Fresh fish skin should gleam like expensive shot silk and feel young and firm to touch. When you push a finger into the fish body, the flesh should spring back with elasticity, not remain collapsed and dented. Scales (if any) should be tight rather than loose. On cutting, the flesh should feel firm and tight, not flabby, waterlogged or flaky. Even fresh fish can be flabby and in poor condition after spawning, so prodding as well as sniffing is important.

Inspect the eyes of fish you are buying. Those of fresh produce are clear, bright, shiny and gleaming. Once the fish starts to deteriorate, the eyes become shrunken and cloudy.

Also check the gills of your potential purchase, which should be a healthy pinky or bright red, not a dingy brown.

It's always best to buy fish whole so you can assess the above features more easily. If you only want fillets or steaks, choose your fish then ask the fishmonger to cut the amount you require. If he doesn't want to do this, the simplest thing is to vote with your feet. I haven't yet met a dedicated fishmonger who doesn't leap proudly to display his wares when a customer expresses interest and a desire to experiment.

When fish is guaranteed ultra-fresh, it is delicious. It is also exceptionally good for health when eaten raw, Japanese-style, as sushi or sashimi.

How Much Fish To Buy

The wastage with fish (through discarding skin, heads, bones, shells) varies but is typically around a third (e.g. monkfish) to a half. As a rule of thumb, flat or round fish have as much skin and bone as edible flesh, so you should always buy double the amount you actually want to eat. With fish that have exceptionally large heads (e.g. John Dory, gurnard), you need to be more generous and allow 680g (1½lb) of fish to obtain 225g (8oz) of usable flesh. The wastage isn't really wasted however – most of it can be boiled with herbs and vegetables to make wonderfully healthy stocks, soups or sauces that will enhance any meal.

Fishy Relations

To whet your appetite for wet fish, I've included a description of the more commonly available fish. I've grouped them according to families so you can get an idea of which fish look and taste similar.

Please resist the temptation to batter your fillets and deep-fry them before serving with chips. They'll all taste the same if you do – and pile on the calories and saturated fats to offset the benefits of their intrinsic oils. The best way to appreciate different fish flavours is by experimenting with simple recipes (*see those provided by Michelle Berriedale-Johnson in Part Three*). You can also try simply poaching fillets in a court-bouillon, or wrapping them in greaseproof (wax) paper or foil with fresh herbs and spring onions (scallions) then baking en papillotte.

THE SALMON FAMILY
Atlantic salmon, Pacific salmon
Salmon is an oily fish whose flesh tends to flakiness and is best slightly undercooked to prevent it becoming gritty and dry. I usually buy salmon fillets rather than steaks as they cook more evenly and any bones are easily removed. Salmon needs to be poached or covered with a light sauce for moistness. If baking with herbs, always wrap salmon in foil to retain the juices. I like to add a dash of white wine to the foil parcel too.

THE HERRING FAMILY

Sardines, anchovies, herring, shad

NB A sardine is a young pilchard. A pilchard is a mature sardine.

The herring family contains exceptionally oily fish. They are a rich source of EPA, which helps to thin the blood, has a beneficial effect on cholesterol levels and discourages hardening of the arteries.

Fresh sardines, of which there are several species, are very different to those encountered crushed in a tin, and are especially nice simply grilled (broiled).

Anchovies are famous for their pungent, salty flavour, which adds a distinctive taste to many Mediterranean dishes. The practice of eating fresh, unsalted anchovies is uncommon in the UK but well worth trying, as most people with high BP need to avoid excess salt. Unsalted anchovies can be split open raw, cleaned and marinated in lemon juice for 24 hours. Serve as an antipasto with drinks – rather like an Italian anchovy gravadlax!

Herring is one of our finest and best-known fish. The Scots cook them by rolling in coarse-cut oatmeal and frying, though grilling (broiling) is a healthier option.

Shad are marred only by their numerous small bones. According to legend, they represent a discontented porcupine turned inside out by a mean-minded spirit. The best time to eat shad is in May as they start swimming up river to spawn.

THE COD FAMILY

Cod, hake, haddock

Cod is the fish that comes closest to a staple in our diet. Specimens weighing over 90kg (200lb) have been recorded, but the usual market weight is around 4.5kg (10lb). The flesh is white with big, chunky flakes and a mild, slightly sweet, if bland flavour. It cries out for a robust, strongly flavoured sauce – using red wine and garlic as a base is ideal.

Hake must be eaten very fresh as its flesh is denser than that of cod and quickly becomes insipid and watery. The whole fish then looks washed out and squashy and falls apart when filleted. Hake is popular poached, steamed or baked and is also used to make fish balls.

Haddock has a stronger flavour and a greyer flesh than cod but also needs a robustly flavoured sauce or plenty of fresh herbs and garlic.

THE PERCH-LIKE FISH

Barracuda, sea bass, sea bream, grouper, red and grey mullet; snapper, parrotfish, weever, wrasse

Barracuda have a devastating array of teeth but taste wonderful chargrilled with garlic, rosemary and marjoram. This fish has a reputation as an aphrodisiac – probably because of its outrageous aggression and virility.

Sea bass is one of my favourite fish with a soft, dense flesh of delicate flavour. Its texture is firm, relatively free of bones and retains its shape well during cooking. Be wary of the spikes on fins and around the gills. Always gut bass as soon as possible as its innards ferment to quickly taint its delicate flesh. Never serve a strongly flavoured sauce with bass or you will drown the gourmet flavour of the flesh.

Sea bream are gorgeous-coloured fish – black or red with distinctive orange stripes. They can be grilled (broiled) or baked whole or filleted – try marinating in fresh herbs and wine before cooking.

Grouper has firm, flaky meat of good flavour. It is a popular fish in the Mediterranean and is now more easily available in the UK.

Red mullet are a glorious crimson tinged with yellow. Their flesh is delicately flavoured, with a hint of lobster, and comes apart in thick, firm flakes. In the Mediterranean, it is usually grilled (broiled), fried or baked. It can also be eaten cooked whole and uncleaned as the liver is a reputed delicacy, lacking the gall-bladder bile that makes so many fish livers bitter.

Grey mullet can be finely flavoured but sometimes taste of mud as these fish are bottom-feeders. For this reason, I usually poach them in a strong stock and sprinkle liberally with garlic and thyme.

Wrasse are an interesting fish as, when sleeping, they experience periods of rapid eye movement (REM) which, in humans, is associated with dreaming! Wrasse tend to be added to stews and soups as their flesh has yellow tones that can be off-putting when cooked alone. Along with their cousin, weaver, wrasse are a basic component of bouillabaisse.

Parrotfish are now often seen in British fishmongers. Its mouth is beaked like a parrot as it gnaws and crunches coral for a pastime – when not sleeping like the wrasse. It is a spectacular fish – rich with reds, pinks, greens, blues and splashes of yellow. Steaming is the recommended method of cooking.

Snappers – named after their well-toothed, active mouths – are mainly from the Caribbean or Asian waters. The bones are easy to find and the flavour is mild and sweet, yet distinctly fishy. The moist, firm flakes absorb flavours from stock very well.

THE MACKEREL FAMILY

Mackerel, tuna, swordfish

I grew up on fresh mackerel caught round the coast of Padstow in Cornwall. It is a handsome fish, iridescent with greens, blues and blacks with a silver-white belly. The cooked flesh is greyish with bands of brown meat near the skin. The flavour is strong and reminiscent of sardines. Because of its high oil content, mackerel goes off quickly. I like it best filleted, sprinkled with flour to absorb the healthy oils, and freshly grilled (broiled) so that the flour gives it a crisp, tasty coating. Liberally douse with lemon juice and serve with a plain, green salad and minty boiled potatoes. Because of its oiliness, mackerel is best complemented by acidic sauces (such as gooseberry, cranberry and rhubarb) or sousing (the Cornish term for pickling) in balsamic vinegar.

Tuna (also known as tunny) is best eaten before it sees the inside of a tin. Tuna are unusual fish as they are warm blooded and have a greater need for oxygen than other fish. In order to obtain this, they must swim constantly at quite a speed to drive water over their gills. As they can never slow down, their musculature is highly developed with a distinctive flavour. Tuna have a firm, heavy meat that flakes easily and tends to be filling. In Japan, it is highly prized raw as a component of sashimi.

Tuna steaks (skipjack and yellowfin are most common) are delicious grilled (broiled) but take care not to overcook and dry them out.

Swordfish has a compact meat with a flavour reminiscent of chicken. It is delicious grilled (broiled) and sprinkled with olive oil, lemon juice, fresh herbs and plenty of black pepper. Make sure the meat is fresh, as frozen swordfish steaks have all the attraction of eating leather.

THE GURNARD FAMILY

Gurnard, redfish, rockfish, scorpion fish

Gurnard can grow larger than the other fish in this family. It has firm, white flesh capable of being filleted, although it is usually cooked whole, stuffed with herbs.

The other fish in this family are suitable only for fish stews and soups. Most are small and have a rather dry flesh. The French call them *rascasse* and they are a requisite for classic bouillabaisse.

THE THIN/FLAT FISH FAMILY

Brill, halibut; John Dory, plaice, sole, turbot

Turbot is an unremarkable-looking, oval flat fish with a speckled, dark back and bony, limpet-like protuberances on its skin – hence its nickname of nail-head. The texture and flavour of fresh turbot is difficult to surpass, however, and it is often served with intricate, delicate, yet exquisite chef's sauces. It even has a cooking pot – the turbotière – especially designed for it. The lovely clear white flesh is firm, moist and succulent. To my mind, it is in the same class as lobster – a treat for that special occasion. Turbot can be steamed, poached, fried, grilled (broiled) or baked en papillote. The head and bones make one of the finest fish stocks.

Brill is similar to turbot with sweet, white meat that is nicely moist.

Halibut can easily weigh over 227kg (500lb) – as much as three average-sized human males! The meat is therefore divided into chunks before it reaches the fishmonger. In the 19th century, halibut was a delicacy when seasoned with freshly grated nutmeg, salt and pepper and baked in the oven. It can be cooked in any of the ways described for firm, white-fleshed fish, and is lovely poached with mushrooms and dill.

John Dory is a remarkable-looking fish – thin-bodied rather than flat with vicious spines and gills. Its profile, head-on, is like a razor's edge so it can creep up on prey without being seen. One black spot adorns each side of the fish which, according to legend, represents St Peter's thumb prints. John Dory has a lovely, firm texture and is delicately flavoured, hence its French name of *poule de mer* – sea chicken. It is one of my favourite fish (especially served with a Cointreau sauce), as long as I can find one large enough to deliver fair-sized fillets. Its large head and gut account for 60 per cent of its weight and, because it is so thin, meat is scarce on small fish. You need to allow 680g (1½lb) of John Dory to obtain 225g (8oz) of usable flesh.

Plaice is one of the best-known flat fish, similar in appearance to flounder but with bony nodules on its head. When fresh, the flavour of plaice is delicate if rather wishy-washy but, unfortunately, it rapidly becomes stale. Some gourmets say plaice is best eaten in the spring, while others shun the fish at that time of year when they are spawning. Plaice feed on bivalves such as cockles and mussels and also forage on the sea floor. The flavour is preferable if they live over sandy bottoms as gravel and mud tend to dull the flavour of the meat and eradicate all traces of sweetness. They can be poached, grilled (broiled) or fried, the later being more common in the UK.

Sole is so-named because the ancient Greeks thought the fish would form an ideal slipper for ocean nymphs. Dover sole is considered the king of sole as the fish is well-suited to being cooked on the bone. The meat remains firm and the skeleton intact, allowing for easy removal on the plate. Lemon sole does not have this distinction – and indeed belongs to a different family. Sandy bottoms also make for firmer, sweeter flesh than mud or gravel sea floors. Slip soles are small Dover sole weighing up to 225g (8oz) each. You would need two per person for a decent-sized meal.

Fish Without True Bones

Monkfish, dogfish, ray, shark, skate

Monkfish is really in a class of its own, but I include it here with the cartilaginous fish as we usually buy the flesh without any bone. Monkfish is more properly called angler fish. It is an ugly beast named after the fishing-rod-like structure with simulated bait that dangles over its mouth. The fish lies well disguised on the sea floor, its rod waving enticingly. As soon as a smaller fish investigates this titbit, the giant jaws attack as the monkfish makes an impressive leap. A 26-inch angler fish has been known to swallow a 23-inch fish whole!

Only the tail of the monkfish is edible. This flesh is firm, pearly white and slightly gelatinous. After spawning, the meat (known as 'slinkfish') is similar to a tasteless milk jelly – so don't forget the prod test.

Monkfish must be eaten fresh and only lightly cooked. If stale or overdone, the flesh rapidly starts to resemble latex rubber. The meat can be poached, steamed, grilled (broiled), fried or even roasted like a leg of lamb. The head, though difficult to obtain, makes an excellent stock.

Many lovers of monkfish claim it resembles lobster meat. Certainly it is used commercially to simulate crab sticks, lobster claws and scampi. Its major advantage is the lack of bones to negotiate. A tough membrane accompanies the tail meat and this is best removed before cooking.

Dogfish (rock salmon, huss) is merely another name for smaller members of the shark family. The skin is like sandpaper and dogfish possess large, volatile intestines which need removing as soon as possible if you are buying the fish intact. Dogfish has a robust flavour and texture. It is well suited to soup or a strongly flavoured sauce.

Fresh shark meat resembles chicken in flavour and texture, while marlin is similar to pork. Forget all you ever learned about sharks perfusing their flesh with urea to offset the osmotic effects of seawater. You honestly wouldn't know – until the meat starts to go stale. Then the smell of ammonia reminiscent of pungent latrines will take your breath away. The shark I've eaten in England has always disappointed, however – it needs to be ultra-fresh before being blackened on the chargrill with fresh herbs and lime to find the most succulent flavours.

Skate and ray should always be eaten fresh – never old or frozen. If you don't believe me, try freezing a piece of wing. When it is defrosted, the flesh will smell so strongly of ammonia, it will knock you over from five paces. I am told, however, that this signals the departure of urea and should be welcomed. Experts say that skate and ray are best eaten a couple of days after death. Rather them than me! When fresh, the white meat peels off the cartilage plates of the wings in delightful, sweet-tasting strips. The classic sauce is a beurre noir flavoured with ghee and capers. I prefer a sauce made from white wine, Greek yoghurt, nutmeg, rosemary and thyme.

Fish Oil Supplements

If you aren't keen on eating more fish, capsules containing omega-3 fish oils are widely available (take 300–3,000mg daily). Natural fish oils contain little vitamin E and can go rancid easily so, if buying fish oil capsules, choose preparations fortified with vitamin E. Some researchers suggest taking 30–200iu of vitamin E and 50–200mcg of selenium daily as well.

Fish oil supplements should be taken only under strict medical supervision if you:

- have a tendency to bleed easily or are taking a blood-thinning agent such as warfarin
- are diabetic – monitor blood glucose levels carefully as control may change.

CHAPTER 6

High Blood Pressure, Folic Acid and Homocysteine

Folic acid is the synthetic form of the naturally occurring vitamin, folate, that is widely found in fruit, green leafy vegetables, nuts, pulses and yeast extracts. Folic acid is absorbed more efficiently from the intestines than naturally occurring folate, and is more readily used by the body. Although it is difficult to obtain optimum levels from natural food sources, supplements and foods fortified with folic acid, such as breakfast cereals, are increasingly available.

Folic acid and folate are both water-soluble and readily lost from the body in urine, so our stores are very low. As a result, a lack of this nutrient in the diet rapidly causes deficiency, and it is believed to be the most widespread vitamin deficiency in developed countries.

Folic acid is involved in a wide number of metabolic reactions, cell division and in protein and sugar metabolism.

Homocysteine

Homocysteine is an amino acid formed in the body from the breakdown of the dietary amino acid, methionine. A raised blood level of homocysteine is now recognized as an important risk factor for developing coronary heart disease and stroke, as it is highly reactive. When it accumulates in the circulation, it causes oxidation damage to the lining of artery walls so they become narrow and inflexible.

As it is so toxic, homocysteine levels are normally tightly controlled by three different enzymes that convert homocysteine to cysteine – a safe end-product used by cells for growth.

Two of the three enzymes that control homocysteine levels depend on folic acid (and to a lesser extent vitamins B6 and B12) for their activity. Those who do not obtain enough folic acid or B-vitamins for optimum enzyme function will have a raised level of homocysteine and, consequently, an increased risk of circulatory problems. A study of 14,000 people in the US found that those with higher than normal homocysteine levels had three times the risk of a heart attack. Unfortunately, lack of folic acid seems to be common – US surveys, for example, suggest that only 40–50 per cent of people obtain enough folic acid from their diet for normal processing of homocysteine.

Genetic mutations can also decrease the activity of any one of the three controlling enzymes to raise homocysteine levels. Around one in ten people are affected, inheriting higher than normal blood levels of homocysteine to triple their risk of these diseases. One in 160,000 people have extremely high levels, with 30 times the risk of premature heart disease and osteoporosis. After the menopause, some women are also less able to process homocysteine so levels build up to increase the risk of osteoporosis and coronary heart disease. It has been estimated that 10 per cent of the risk of coronary artery disease in the general population is, in fact, due to homocysteine.

The risks associated with an elevated homocysteine level are therefore comparable to those of an abnormally raised cholesterol level. However, it is easier to correct a high homocysteine level through dietary intervention. Taking a vitamin and mineral supplement providing as little as 200mcg of folic acid per day (the EC RDA) is effective in lowering moderately raised plasma homocysteine levels. High levels of homocysteine can be reduced by taking folic acid supplements supplying 400–650mcg per day. People with a family or personal history of coronary heart disease may wish to consider taking supplements of at least 400mcg folic acid daily.

In the UK, some food packagings have special flashes to show they contain folic acid – these were designed for pregnant women whose need for folic acid is significantly raised, but are also helpful for people with increased risk of heart disease. Products flashed *Contains Folic Acid* can provide at least one-sixth of the average daily requirement, while those flashed *With Extra Folic Acid* are enriched to provide at least half the average daily requirement.

Folic acid should usually be taken together with vitamin B12. This is because lack of vitamin B12 (which leads to damage of the nervous system, especially the spinal cord) is masked by taking folic acid supplements (as this prevents the occurrence of pernicious anaemia which usually allows lack of vitamin B12 to be detected).

CHAPTER 7

High Blood Pressure and Salt

All your cells are bathed in a fluid containing a variety of dissolved chemicals and salts. Once dissolved, these separate into particles known as ions that carry an electric charge. Common table salt – known chemically as sodium chloride – dissolves to form two types of particle:

- sodium ions that carry a positive electric charge (Na+)
- chloride ions that carry a negative electric charge (Cl^-).

Sodium is the main positively charged ion found in the fluid bathing the outside of body cells but is present inside cells only in low concentrations. This is because a special salt pump found in all cell membranes moves sodium out of cells by swapping it for potassium ions, which also carry a single positive electric charge (K+).

	Sodium ions (Na+)	Potassium ions (K+)
Amount found inside cells	9%	90%
Amount found outside cells	91%	10%

The Sodium–Potassium Pump

The sodium–potassium pump forces sodium out of your cells by swapping it for potassium, which is forced inside your cells. The sodium–potassium pump transports three positively charged sodium ions out of a cell for every two positively charged potassium ions it transports in. It is therefore an electrogenic (electricity-producing) pump as it produces a net movement of positive charge out of each cell. As a result of these ion changes, the inside of the cell is negatively charged compared with the outside of the cell, and there is a potential difference across the membrane of most – if not all – living cells.

Table: Concentration of various ions inside and outside a spinal nerve

ION	Concentration inside cell	Concentration outside cell
Sodium (Na+)	15mmol/l	150mmol/l
Chloride (Cl-)	9mmol/l	125mmol/l
Potassium (K+)	150mmol/l	5.5mmol/l

Interestingly, the active transport of sodium and potassium ions in and out of cells is one of the main energy-using metabolic processes occurring within the body. It is estimated to account for 33 per cent of energy (in the form of glucose fuel) used by cells overall, and 70 per cent of energy used by nerve cells alone.

Sodium and High Blood Pressure

Common salt therefore plays an important role in cell functions, and a certain amount of sodium is essential for good health. However, researchers now believe that the rise in blood pressure seen with increasing age is directly linked to your lifetime's intake of excessive dietary salt (sodium chloride). In fact, some experts would say that hypertension developing in younger adults is just an early exaggeration of the sodium-induced rise in blood pressure that normally occurs with increasing age. Certainly, data from the Intersalt study (involving 10,000 people in 32 countries) suggest the link between salt intake and rising blood pressure with increasing age may be stronger than previously thought.

Not everyone, however, is sensitive to the effects of salt. The interaction between someone's salt intake and their genetic predisposition to hypertension is poorly understood. Researchers have recently discovered a gene that they believe may be associated with an increased risk of inheriting salt sensitivity. It is estimated that at least one in two people are genetically programmed to develop high blood pressure if their intake of salt (sodium chloride) is excessive. Although not everyone is sensitive to this effect, it is worth cutting back on salt if you suffer from hypertension. Researchers have also found that people with the highest blood levels of the kidney hormone, renin, are most likely to respond to a low-sodium, high-potassium diet. If you suffer from kidney problems as well as hypertension, you should definitely follow a low-salt diet as you may not be able to excrete as much salt as normally, allowing it to build up in your body and contribute to your blood pressure problems.

Everyone with high blood pressure should consider lowing their salt intake. Ideally, you should obtain between 4–6g of salt per day. Average intakes, however, are 6g per day with some people eating as much as 12g of salt daily. Reducing salt intake by 3g per day from 9g to 6g is estimated to lower your risk of a stroke by 22 per cent and your risk of death from CHD by 16 per cent.

Unfortunately, most dietary salt (around 75 per cent) is in the form of hidden salt added to processed foods including canned products, ready-prepared meals, biscuits, cakes and breakfast cereals. This means that without checking labels of bought products and avoiding those containing high amounts of salt, it is difficult to influence your salt intake as much as is desirable to reduce your risk of hypertension.

To cut back on salt intake avoid:

* adding salt during cooking or at the table
* obviously salty foods such as crisps, bacon, salted nuts
* tinned products, especially those canned in brine
* cured, smoked or pickled fish/meats
* meat pastes, pâtés
* ready-prepared meals
* packet soups and sauces
* stock cubes and yeast extracts.

Where salt is essential, use mineral-rich rock salt rather than table salt, or use a low-sodium brand of salt sparingly. Salt is easily replaceable with herbs and spices as it doesn't take long to re-train your taste buds. Adding lime juice to food stimulates taste buds and decreases the amount of salt you need, too.

Studies suggest that not adding salt during cooking or at the table will lower your systolic blood pressure by at least 5mmHg. If everyone did this, it is estimated that the incidence of stroke in the population would be reduced by as much as 26 per cent and coronary heart disease by 15 per cent.

NB When checking labels, those giving salt content as sodium need to be multiplied by 2.5 to give true salt content: for example, a serving of soup containing 0.4g sodium contains 1g salt.

Potassium

Potassium is the main positively charged electrolyte found inside your cells, where it balances the sodium ions found in the fluid outside your cells. Potassium is essential for muscle contraction, nerve conduction and for the production of nucleic acids, proteins and energy. As far as blood pressure is concerned, potassium is important in that it helps to flush excess sodium out of the body through the kidneys. The sodium–potassium pump in the walls of kidney tubules can swap potassium ions for sodium ions as discussed above. Because the body swaps sodium for potassium in this way, a diet low in potassium is linked with a higher risk of high blood pressure and stroke – especially if your diet is also high in sodium. In one study, people taking anti-hypertensive medication were able to reduce their drug dose by half (under medical supervision) after increasing the potassium content of their food.

Ideally, you need to obtain around 3,500mg of potassium per day. Most people get less than this, however, as the average intake is around 3,187mg. Some people obtain as little as 1,700mg of potassium from their food. To increase your potassium intake, eat more:

* seafood
* fresh fruit, especially bananas, dried apricots, tomatoes and pears
* fruit juices and fruit yoghurts
* vegetables, especially mushrooms, potatoes, aubergines (eggplant), peppers, squash and spinach
* pulses such as peas and lima beans
* wholegrain breakfast cereals (check labels for sodium chloride content).

Steam rather than boil vegetables to retain more of their mineral content. If you do boil vegetables, keep the water to make gravy or a low-fat sauce afterwards.

In general, fresh whole foods are a good source of potassium and contain little sodium (e.g. freshly squeezed orange juice), while processed foods (e.g. orange cordial) usually contain little potassium but lots of sodium.

Low-salt products containing potassium chloride to replace sodium chloride are popular but can taste bitter. Too much potassium can, unfortunately, be harmful too, so the best way to ensure adequate but safe supplies is to eat potassium-rich foods.

Chapter 8

High Blood Pressure, Fruit and Vegetables

Fruit, vegetables, nuts, seeds and pulses are rich sources of vitamins, minerals, fibre and at least 20 non-nutrient substances, known as phytochemicals, that have a beneficial effect on health. Some of these substances are powerful antioxidants, while others have beneficial hormone-like actions or anti-inflammatory effects in the body.

Sources of Phytochemicals

Many studies suggest that those who eat the most raw and fresh fruit (including tomatoes) are least likely to develop coronary heart disease and cancer. The exact reason is unknown, but is likely to be due to a variety of beneficial substances found in fruit. These are described below.

FLAVONOIDS

These natural antioxidants help to maintain health and protect against disease. As antioxidants, they protect cell membranes from damage, and also help to prevent hardening and furring up of the arteries. Almost every fruit and vegetable contains flavonoids, of which over 20,000 are known to exist. One study found that men who ate the most flavonoids had less than half the number of fatal heart attacks compared with those who ate the least. The chief sources of flavonoids in the study were apples, onions and tea.

SOLUBLE FIBRE

This helps to keep the bowels working normally. A number of studies have found that those eating more fruit are less likely to suffer from cancer of the colon. Fibre also has beneficial effects on the absorption of dietary fat.

MICRONUTRIENTS

These contain all the important vitamins, minerals and trace elements you need. They are good sources of the antioxidant vitamins C, E, betacarotene and mineral selenium. Fruit also contains potassium, which helps to flush excess sodium through the kidneys and may help to reduce high blood pressure.

PHYTOCHEMICALS

These plant chemicals seem to help protect against cancer by blocking enzymes needed for the growth of cancer cells.

PHYTOESTROGENS

These plant hormones have a weak oestrogen-like effect in the body. There are three main types – isoflavones, flavonoids and lignans. The isoflavones are the most widely studied and are useful for both men and women as they interact with oestrogen receptors within the circulation to mimic some of the beneficial effects of oestrogen. These include helping to dilate coronary arteries, increase heart function, reduce blood levels of harmful LDL-cholesterol and reduce blood stickiness to prevent unwanted clotting. These findings may help explain why the Japanese – who eat up to 100 times more isoflavones than are found in the Western diet – have one of the lowest rates of coronary heart disease in the world.

Phytoestrogens also have beneficial antioxidant and anti-inflammatory actions, which may reduce the risk of atherosclerosis. Soya beans are a rich source of isoflavones and, based on scientific evidence from over 50 independent studies, the US Food and Drug Administration (FDA) stated in October 1999 that it will authorize health claims on food labels that 'A diet low in saturated fat and cholesterol, and which includes 25g soya protein per day, can significantly reduce the risk of coronary heart disease.' Soya is also a rich source of protein, calcium and fibre.

Nuts

Walnuts are a rich source of omega-3 oils and can lower a high cholesterol level and reduce the risk of coronary heart disease. Walnuts contain a high ratio of monounsaturated and polyunsaturated to saturated fats. Compared to most other nuts, which contain monounsaturated fatty acids, walnuts are unique because they are rich in both omega-6 (linoleic) and omega-3 (linolenic) polyunsaturated fatty acids. In fact, 12 per cent of their total fat content is the essential linolenic acid, which cannot be made in the body. They also contain useful amounts of vitamin B, folate, antioxidant polyphenols and vitamin E.

Although walnuts are energy-rich (60g supply 578 calories), dietary intervention studies show that eating walnuts does not cause a net gain in body weight when they are eaten as a replacement food.

A recent analysis of five clinical trials involving around 200 people consistently found that walnuts lowered blood cholesterol concentrations when included in a heart-healthy diet. In one study, nine healthy males added 84g of walnuts to their daily diet for four weeks and reduced their total blood cholesterol level by 12 per cent more than a control group not eating walnuts. Even more importantly, harmful LDL-cholesterol levels were reduced by 16 per cent. Studies using almonds and hazelnuts also revealed beneficial effects on blood lipid profiles.

In another trial looking at the effects of eating walnuts on blood lipids and blood pressure, 18 healthy males followed two mixed natural diets for four weeks. Both diets conformed to the National Cholesterol Education Program and contained identical foods and macronutrients. In one diet, however, 20 per cent of calories were derived from walnuts, and offset by eating lesser amounts of fatty foods, meat, oils, margarine and butter. When following the walnut diet for four weeks, the average total cholesterol level was 22.4mg per decilitre lower than when the same men followed the non-walnut, cholesterol-lowering diet. Levels of LDL- and HDL-cholesterol were 18.2mg per decilitre and 2.3mg per decilitre lower respectively. These represented reductions of 12.4 per cent total cholesterol, 16.3 per cent LDL-cholesterol and 4.9 per cent HDL-cholesterol. Although the average blood-pressure values did not change throughout the study, walnuts would still appear to be beneficial as, by lowering the relative levels of LDL-cholesterol, they can help to reduce the development of atherosclerosis and future complications of hypertension such as a heart attack. Other studies have confirmed an inverse relationship between nut consumption and risk of coronary heart disease.

It is best to buy walnuts in shells or vacuum packs as exposure to air rapidly reduces their nutrient value. Most people eat less than 4g of walnuts per week. Increasing your intake to 28g per day would help to decrease blood LDL-cholesterol levels by 6 per cent.

What is a Serving?

The benefits of eating more fruit and vegetables – at least five servings per day, and preferably eight to ten – are so great that some experts now feel we should recommend increased intakes of antioxidants from fruit, vegetables, green and black tea and red wine (in moderation), rather than advocating a diet low in cholesterol and saturated fat.

A serving, or portion, of fruit and vegetables is basically the amount you are happy to eat in one sitting – the more the better. Typically, this would amount to:

- a glass of fruit juice
- a large mixed salad
- 1 large beef tomato or 2 medium tomatoes
- a handful of grapes, cherries or berries
- a single apple, orange, kiwi, peach, pear, nectarine or banana
- ½ grapefruit, ½ ogen melon, ½ mango, ½ papaya
- 2–4 dates, figs, satsumas, passion fruit, apricots, plums or prunes
- a handful of nuts
- a generous helping of green or root vegetables (excluding potatoes).

CHAPTER 9

High Blood Pressure and Garlic

Garlic (*Allium sativum*) is such a popular culinary herb that, worldwide, average consumption is equivalent to one clove per person a day. It has been cultivated for millennia and has a number of medicinal uses, being antioxidant, antiseptic, antibacterial and antiviral. The evidence that garlic lowers blood cholesterol levels and blood pressure is now overwhelming, and its most important use relates to its ability to maintain a healthy circulation and reduce the risk of coronary heart disease (CHD) and stroke.

The main substance derived from garlic that protects against coronary heart disease is allicin, which gives a crushed clove its characteristic smell. Allicin is not present in whole garlic cloves, however, which contain an odourless precursor called alliin – an amino acid unique to the garlic family. Alliin is stored within garlic cells, separated from the enzyme (alliinase) designed to break it down. It is only when alliin and alliinase come together that beneficial allicin (diallyl thiosulphinate) is made. This natural reaction occurs as soon as a clove of garlic is cut or crushed and releases its characteristic odour.

Allicin prevents cells from taking up cholesterol, reduces cholesterol production in the liver and hastens excretion of fatty acids, thereby discouraging atherosclerosis. Sulphur compounds formed by the degradation of allicin are also beneficial and are incorporated into long-chain fatty acid molecules, to act as antioxidants. Antioxidants protect blood LDL-cholesterol molecules against oxidation and reduce their uptake by scavenger cells to protect against atherosclerosis.

Garlic and the Circulatory System

Garlic powder extracts can lower blood pressure enough to reduce the risk of a stroke by up to 40 per cent. At daily doses of 600–900mg, for periods of between 28 and 180 days, systolic BP was reduced in studies by an average of 8 per cent (and up to 17 per cent) while diastolic BP was reduced by an average of 12 per cent (and up to 16 per cent). This reduction is a gradual process, occurring with a minimum of two to three months' treatment. These findings are significant, as a reduction of just 5mmHg in diastolic pressure has been shown to reduce the risk of CHD by as much as 16 per cent. As garlic extracts usually do better than this, they have been estimated to lower the risk of CHD by a massive 38 per cent through their action on blood pressure alone.

This effect is thought to be due to a combination of increasing the fluidity of blood (i.e. decreasing its stickiness), a beneficial effect on the way sodium and potassium ions cross cell membranes, and dilation of blood vessels by relaxing smooth muscle cells. The blood vessel dilation effect can be seen within five hours after taking a single dose.

Garlic has other beneficial effects against the risk of CHD. Clinical trials using standardized extracts have shown that people taking the equivalent of 800mg dried garlic powder per day experience an average fall in blood cholesterol level of 12 per cent after four months' therapy. Triglycerides, another form of fatty acids found in the blood, fall by around 13 per cent.

One of the first events that trigger atherosclerosis is the accumulation of platelets (blood-clotting cell fragments) on damaged parts of the arterial wall. At later stages, platelet aggregation and clot (thrombus) build-up hastens furring up and narrowing of arteries. By inhibiting this platelet clumping, taking garlic regularly can protect against both the first and later stages of atherosclerosis. Platelet clumping is significantly decreased after a dose equivalent to half a clove of garlic and lasts for three hours. Some of the ingredients in garlic (ajoene, methylallyl trisulphide and dimethyl trisulphide) seem to be as potent as aspirin in this respect.

Studies suggest that garlic therapy improves the circulation by increasing blood flow through small arteries (arterioles) and small veins (venules). Garlic dilates the arterioles by an average of 4.2 per cent and the venules by 5.9 per cent. As a result, garlic can improve blood flow to the skin by almost 50 per cent (helpful for Raynaud's disease and for chilblains) and to the nail folds by as much as 55 per cent. Another interesting study found that taking garlic extracts increased the elasticity of the aorta so the heart had to work less hard to pump blood out into the body. These effects all help to lower peripheral resistance so that blood pressure falls.

Garlic improves blood fluidity by increasing the levels of a natural clot-busting reaction, fibrinolysis, by at least 25 per cent. In one study, fibrinolytic activity was increased by 70 per cent within a few hours of taking raw garlic. This effect seems to be most pronounced in those with CHD – perhaps because their lipid metabolism is more abnormal in the first place. It also decreases blood stickiness, decreases blood-cell clumping and improves blood fluidity.

For people who suffer from calf pain on walking more than 100 yards due to reduced blood flow to the legs (intermittent claudication), taking garlic for just three months has been shown to increase the distance that can be walked before calf pain starts by as much as 30 per cent.

An important recent study followed 152 patients for over 4 years and found that garlic tablets could reduce and even reverse hardening and furring up of the arteries (atherosclerosis). In those not taking garlic tablets, atherosclerotic plaques built up by 15.6 per cent over the four years, while in those taking garlic, plaque volume decreased by 2.6 per cent – a combined difference of 18.2 per cent. Due to all these beneficial effects on the circulation, taking garlic extracts is estimated to reduce the risk of a heart attack by 50 per cent.

All these beneficial effects on the circulation can be demonstrated within five hours of taking a single dose of 600–900mg of garlic (supplying 1,000–1,500mcg allicin). The effects are dose related and wear off over 24 hours. Garlic has such a powerful medicinal action that, in Germany, garlic powder tablets containing the equivalent of 4g of fresh cloves are available on prescription to treat high blood cholesterol levels and high blood pressure.

Garlic and General Health

As well as providing considerable protection against CHD, most people also notice an improvement in their general wellbeing when taking garlic. One study assessed people's psychological state before and after four months' treatment with standardized garlic extracts. There was a marked improvement in positive mood characteristics (activity, elated mood, concentration, sensitivity) and a drop in negative mood characteristics (anxiety, irritation) in those taking garlic tablets, compared with no significant change in those taking an inactive placebo.

Large doses of fresh garlic (7 to 28 cloves per day) would have a similar effect but would be unpalatable and antisocial. Garlic tablets are available with a special enteric coating so their odour is much less apparent during treatment. Include garlic in your diet as much as possible, but consider taking a daily garlic supplement as well.

NB Garlic supplements often contain concentrated garlic extracts, so the milligrams supplied may seem lower than those quoted here for unconcentrated dried garlic. In these cases, check allicin content and aim for one supplying at least 1,000mcg allicin daily.

CHAPTER 10

High Blood Pressure and Tea

Tea is one of the most popular drinks in the world. An ancient Chinese legend claims tea was discovered as a beverage in 2737 BC when leaves from a camellia bush fell into the Emperor's cup of hot water. The earliest confirmed reference to the cultivation, processing and drinking of tea is in a Chinese dictionary dating from the fourth century AD.

Tea was first introduced to Europe by the Dutch East India Company in 1610 (around the same time as both coffee and chocolate). We now each drink an average of 3.5 cups per day. The Chinese have long considered tea to be a medicinal beverage, and now we in the West are discovering its beneficial effects on our health.

Green and black tea are similar in that both are made from the young leaves and leaf buds of the same shrub, *Camellia sinensis*. Two main varieties are used: the small-leaved China tea plant (*C. sinensis sinensis*) and the large-leaved Assam tea plant (*C. sinensis assamica*). Green tea is made by steaming and drying fresh tea leaves immediately after harvesting, while black tea is made by crushing and fermenting freshly cut tea leaves so they oxidize before drying. This allows natural enzymes in the tea leaves to produce the characteristic red-brown colour and reduced astringency.

Over 30 per cent of the dry weight of green tea leaves consists of powerful flavonoid antioxidants such as catechins. Green tea extracts appear to have an antioxidant action at least 100 times more powerful than vitamin C, and 25 times more powerful than vitamin E. These are converted into less active antioxidants during fermentation (such as theaflavins and thearubigins) but even so, drinking four to five cups of black tea per day still provides over 50 per cent of the total dietary intake of flavonoid antioxidants (other sources include fruit and vegetables, especially apples and onions). Tea is also a rich source of phytochemicals, the trace element, manganese, and is one of the few natural sources of fluoride, which helps to protect against tooth decay.

Drinking either green or black tea has beneficial effects on blood pressure, blood lipids, blood stickiness and can decrease the risk of coronary heart disease and stroke. Research suggests that those drinking at least four cups of tea a day are half as likely to have a heart attack as non-tea drinkers (its antioxidants reduce oxidation of LDL-cholesterol so less is deposited in artery walls) and less likely to suffer from high blood pressure. High intakes (8 to 10 cups per day) may also reduce the risk of some cancers, especially those of the stomach, colon, rectum, pancreas, breast, skin and bladder. Antioxidants found in green tea extracts are also known to increase resistance to infection, and to protect against premature ageing – hence they are now added to a variety of skin-care preparations.

If you have high blood pressure, aim to drink four cups of green (or black) tea daily, or consider taking green tea extracts. Of the tea consumed worldwide, 20 per cent is taken as green tea, mainly in Asia, while 80 per cent is drunk as black tea, mainly in the West. As green tea is an acquired taste, some people prefer to drink a blend of black and green teas, or to take green tea extracts.

Drinking three to four cups of tea per day, made with semi-skimmed milk, typically provides the following percentage of our daily needs:

- 45 per cent manganese
- 25 per cent vitamin B2
- 16 per cent calcium
- 10 per cent folic acid
- 10 per cent zinc
- 9 per cent potassium
- 9 per cent vitamin B1
- 6 per cent vitamin B5
- 6 per cent vitamin B6
- 5 per cent selenium.

Tea contains a relatively low amount of caffeine compared with coffee, and the health benefits of drinking tea probably outweigh the risks. If you prefer to avoid caffeine, however, a South African tea that is naturally free of caffeine (Redbush or rooibos tea) is a useful alternative.

CHAPTER 11

High Blood Pressure and Red Wine

Lovers of red wine have the ultimate vin-dication: an apparent *carte blanche* to imbibe to their heart's content. The US Food and Drug Administration has allowed vintners to label red wines as good for the health. Many studies around the world have found that a moderate intake of alcohol (20–30g per day) reduces the risk of coronary heart disease by as much as 40 per cent. Red wine, especially with meals, seems particularly beneficial if drunk on a daily basis. One expert has even stated that, as far as coronary heart disease goes: 'A half bottle of good red wine with lunch may be a better preventative medicine than all the cholesterol guidelines combined. Alcohol is a drug that should be used regularly, but at moderate doses of 20–30g per day.'

Comforting words – but the alcohol content of wine may not be the sole explanation for these cardio-protective effects. Red wine contains many compounds whose antioxidant properties play an important role. In fact, non-alcoholic red wine and red grape juice may offer similar protection against coronary heart disease.

Interest in wine initially arose because of the so-called French paradox. Compared with Britain and the US, the French ate as much saturated fat, had similar high cholesterol levels, smoked as much (if not more), took as little exercise and drank lots more wine, yet their risk of CHD was lower than that of any other industrialized country except Japan (where people are protected by their high intake of omega-3 fish oils and soy isoflavones). *Le paradoxe Français* was most evident in Gascony, home of the fatty *saucisses de Toulouse* and the ultimate cardiologists' nightmare – pâté de foie gras.

A decade ago, researchers found that, in Toulouse, the male CHD mortality rate was 78 per 100,000 (women 11 per 100,000) and wine intake averaged half a bottle per day. Some males drank as much as a litre of red wine per day, but always to wash down meals. It was hardly ever drunk on its own. At the same time, in Glasgow, a city not renowned for its love of red wine, the annual male CHD mortality rate was more than four times greater at 380 per 100,000. For women, there was a staggering 12-fold increase in incidence (132 per 100,000). Most males drank lager, beer or spirits and did not take their alcohol with meals.

There was no adequate explanation for this French paradox, though red wine consumption was increasingly thought to play a role.

Red Wine Versus Other Sources of Alcohol

In one large study involving 129,000 people, researchers looked at the usual alcohol preference of the participants who died – wine, spirits or beer. After taking into account the number of drinks consumed per day, a preference for wine was associated with a significantly lower risk of cardio-vascular death (a 30 per cent reduction for men and a 40 per cent reduction for women) when compared with spirit drinkers. This suggested that components other than alcohol might be involved. Another study found that, in 17 countries where wine consumption was known, wine was the only foodstuff with a significant negative correlation with mortality, indicating a protective effect.

The Properties of Red Wine

Wine is a complex liquid containing many substances known to have an antioxidant action, including phenolic compounds such as flavonoids, flavonols, catechins, anthocyanins and soluble tannins. These help to neutralize the free radicals produced as a result of general metabolism, and which are thought to oxidize low-density cholesterol and hasten narrowing and hardening of the arteries (*see page 155*).

Research has shown that the phenolic compounds found in red wine are able to inhibit the oxidation of LDL-cholesterol significantly more than does vitamin E, and that they also inhibit blood clotting (thrombosis), both of which help to reduce the development of atherosclerosis. Red wine also contains procyanidins at concentrations of up to 1gm/l. These polyphenols are also powerful antioxidants and free-radical scavengers.

Another beneficial group of chemicals in red wine are phytoalexins – natural antifungal agents found in the skins of grapes – such as resveratrol. As the making of red wine involves macerating grape skins for longer than when making white wines or champagne, red wine therefore has a much higher concentration. Resveratrol has been shown to help raise levels of protective HDL-cholesterol as well as inhibiting platelet aggregation and clot formation in laboratory tests.

ANTI-PLATELET ACTIVITY

Platelets are small cell fragments in the blood and active components in the clotting process. Some chemicals, such as dietary saturated fats, promote platelet aggregation and the formation of blood clots by making platelets sticky, while others, such as marine fish oils and olive oil, discourage clotting and decrease the likelihood of unwanted thromboses. Inhibition of platelet activity may be one explanation for the French paradox as pilot studies have demonstrated that platelet reactivity is lower in people living in France than those living in Scotland. Another explanation is that, because red wine is mostly consumed with meals, it is absorbed more slowly. This will prolong any protective effect on blood platelets at a time when they are under the influence of dietary saturated fats, which are known to increase their activity. It also helps to protect dietary saturated fats from oxidation so they are less likely to contribute to the athero-sclerotic process.

Beneficial Effects of Alcohol

Much evidence suggests that moderate drinkers (two to three units of alcohol per day) have lower blood pressure, less risk of a stroke, a protective HDL:LDL cholesterol ratio (except in the case of the French paradox) and reduced risk of serious atherosclerosis as well as a lower incidence of coronary heart disease. In moderation, alcohol also counteracts the effects of stress by promoting relaxation – but only at levels of alcohol consumption compatible with health.

Deleterious Effects of Alcohol

Unfortunately, the beneficial effects of alcohol must be weighed against the bad. The key is moderation. Men who regularly drink six units of alcohol per day (e.g. six glasses of wine or three pints of normal-strength beer) or who binge-drink at weekends, have almost twice the risk of sudden cardiovascular death, due to heart-rhythm abnormalities, than moderate or non-drinkers.

Heavy drinkers have an increased risk of death from several conditions, including road traffic accidents, suicide, homicide, certain malignancies, stroke, heart-rhythm disturbances, weakened heart muscle (cardiomyopathy) and cirrhosis of the liver. The incidence of liver disease in France is around twice that in the US and, although it accounts for only three per cent of French deaths, this effect must be borne in mind.

Safe maximum alcohol intakes per week remain at:
14 units for women and 21 units for men.

A weekly intake of over 35 units for women and over 50 units for men is considered dangerous.
1 unit of alcohol = 10g alcohol
= 100ml wine (one small glass)
= 50ml sherry (one measure)
= 25ml spirit (one tot)
= 300ml beer (½ pint)

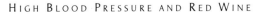

PART THREE

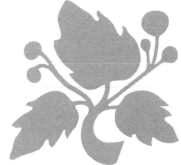

The Recipes

CHAPTER 12

Introduction

As you will know from reading the book this far, controlling your weight and your intake of salt are two of the most important factors that influence your blood pressure. If you can also manage to increase your intake of fresh fruits and vegetables and certain key nutrients – potassium, vitamins C and D, essential fatty acids – your diet will be making a substantial contribution first to lowering, and then to controlling, your blood pressure.

Weight

Although butter, cream and sugar do appear in the following recipes, they do so only in small amounts. This means that you retain flavour but keep the calories down. All the recipes use copious amounts of fresh fruit and vegetables – indeed, many of the dessert and baking recipes do not use any sugar at all, getting their sweetness entirely from fresh and dried fruit. None the less, most of the recipes are pretty filling so you will not be craving a forbidden snack.

Salt

The vast majority of the salt in our diets comes from ready-prepared foods. Not just the packets of crisps or salted peanuts but the lasagnes and moussakas, the breakfast cereals and sometimes even biscuits and cakes. No doubt you have already become an avid 'label reader'.

Never add salt automatically to any dish you are cooking – with the exception of a little in the water in which you cook your pasta! Many of these recipes use seaweeds, herbs and spices to add flavour so you should not need any salt.

The golden rule is not to banish salt from the kitchen but to taste *before* you add the salt, not afterwards. If you do decide to add salt to a dish, add a little less than you think it needs. Our taste buds have become dulled by years of over-salted foods and it takes them a little time to readjust. After a couple of months you will wonder how you could ever have salted food so heavily.

There are also a number of excellent low-sodium salts around – some of them natural sea salts and some ground seaweeds, so it is worth experimenting. These include:

* LoSalt – available in supermarkets
* Solo low-sodium sea salt – available in supermarkets. www.soloseasalt.com
* Seagreens (seaweed flavouring) – available in health-food stores. www.seagreens.com

Potassium

As you are probably aware, potassium is needed to flush excess sodium out of the body – but people with high blood pressure often eat diets low in potassium. Fortunately, potassium is easy to get from foods as most fruits and vegetables contain reasonable amounts, as do pulses, nuts and seafoods. Caffeine addicts will also be relieved to know that coffee is a good source of potassium.

Essential Fatty Acids

It is now widely recognized that 21st-century diets do not include anywhere near enough omega-3 fatty acids. The body cannot manufacture these fatty acids, and we need them to maintain cell structures and arterial walls, among many other things. Fatty acids seem to be helpful in treating high blood pressure and high cholesterol.

Once again, they are not difficult to find in food, the richest sources being nuts and seeds, seed oils and oily fish. You will find that the recipes make copious use of both nuts and seeds, which also add texture and flavour to a wide range of dishes.

Calcium, Magnesium and Vitamin D

Calcium and magnesium work together to maintain bones, teeth and the integrity of cells. Low intakes, especially of magnesium, have been linked to high blood pressure. Vitamin D is needed to help absorb the calcium.

Fortunately, many of the fruits and vegetables (especially the green leafy ones) from which you can get your potassium are also rich in calcium and magnesium. Nuts, seeds, soya beans and oats are also good sources of magnesium – as is bitter chocolate! Root vegetables, dairy products and bony fish (such as sardines and pilchards) are good sources of calcium.

Vitamin D comes from sunlight and from the oily fish you should be eating to boost your levels of essential fatty acids.

Vitamin C

People with high blood pressure tend to have low levels of vitamin C, one of the most important antioxidant vitamins. Fortunately, once again, vitamin C is to be found in exactly the same fruits and vegetables (especially the green leafy ones) you will already be eating to boost your intake of calcium, magnesium and potassium.

Nutrient Content of Recipes

For each of the recipes, you will see that we have given a guide to their nutritional content in the context of high blood pressure. Not all recipes are particularly high in the nutrient concerned but all contain a useful amount.

You will soon learn to recognize foods which are particularly useful, but as a general rule of thumb, any dish containing substantial amounts of nuts, seeds, green leafy vegetables or oily fish will provide you with generous helpings of calcium, magnesium and potassium; anything with lots of nuts, seeds or oily fish will provide generous helpings of essential fatty acids; and all fruits and vegetables, especially when raw, will provide lots of vitamin C.

Happy cooking – happy eating – and good health!

MICHELLE BERRIEDALE-JOHNSON

CHAPTER 13

Soups and Starters

Spinach, Seaweed and Butter Bean Soup

Source of: calcium, magnesium, vitamin C, potassium, EFAs
Dried sea vegetables are now fairly easy to find in good health-food stores – they are very tasty and allow you to dispense with extra salt.

Ingredients

METRIC (IMPERIAL)		AMERICAN
2 tablespoons	rapeseed or olive oil	2 tablespoons
2 medium	leeks, very finely sliced	2 medium
2 tablespoons	mixed dried sea vegetables/salad	2 tablespoons
200g (7oz)	fresh spinach, roughly chopped or frozen chopped spinach, well defrosted	4 cups
1 litre (1¾ pints)	water	4½ cups
1 heaped teaspoon	miso or low-salt vegetable stock cube	1 heaping teaspoon
1 x 395g (14oz) tin	butter beans, drained	1 x 14oz can

Method

1 Cook the leeks very gently in the oil until soft.
2 Add the sea vegetables, the spinach, the water and the miso/vegetable stock.
3 Bring to the boil, cover and simmer gently for 30 minutes until the vegetables are quite cooked and the flavours amalgamated.
4 Add the butter beans and continue to cook for a further 5 minutes before serving.
5 For a smoother soup, purée it in a food processor once it is cooked.

North-African Lentil Soup with Garlic

Source of: calcium, vitamin C, EFAs
A splendidly aromatic soup. Serve hot, sprinkled with chopped fresh coriander (cilantro) or with the warm croutons. Avoid the croutons if you are trying to lose weight as they will have absorbed a lot of oil and therefore be calorific.

Ingredients

SERVES 6

METRIC (IMPERIAL)		AMERICAN
2 tablespoons	sunflower, rapeseed or olive oil	2 tablespoons
4 large	cloves garlic, peeled and sliced	4 large
1 large stick	celery, chopped	1 large stalk
2 heaped teaspoons	ground cumin	2 heaping teaspoons
370g (13oz)	red lentils	2 cups
2 litres (3½ pints)	low-salt vegetable stock or water with	8 cups
	2 teaspoons of miso	
	freshly ground black pepper	
1 handful	fresh coriander (cilantro) leaves, chopped (optional)	1 handful

Croutons:

8–10 tablespoons	sunflower, rapeseed or olive oil	8–10 tablespoons
3	cloves garlic, crushed	3
3 slices	brown bread, cut in small cubes	3 slices

Method

1 Put the oil in a deep pan with the garlic and celery and cook gently for 5–10 minutes or until the vegetables are softening.
2 Add the cumin and the lentils and continue to cook for a few more minutes, then add the liquid and a little seasoning.
3 Bring to the boil and simmer gently for 45–60 minutes or until the lentils have all but disintegrated.
4 Purée the soup in a food processor then return to the pan. Season with freshly ground black pepper to taste – you should not need any extra salt.

Croutons:
1 While the lentils are cooking, heat the oil in a wide frying pan (skillet).
2 Add the garlic and cook gently for several minutes or until lightly cooked through.
3 Increase the heat and add the bread cubes. Fry briskly for 5–6 minutes until the cubes are all well browned but not burnt.
4 Remove from the pan onto kitchen paper to drain off any excess oil.

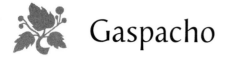

Gaspacho

Source of: vitamin C, potassium, EFAs
A classic gaspacho – very cooling on a hot afternoon.

Ingredients

METRIC (IMPERIAL)		AMERICAN
900g (2lb)	ripe tomatoes, roughly chopped	5 cups
3 large	cloves garlic, peeled and roughly chopped	3 large
1 small	onion, finely chopped	1 small
3 tablespoons	sunflower, rapeseed or olive oil	3 tablespoons
285ml (10fl oz)	dry white wine	1⅓ cups
570ml (1 pint)	low-salt chicken stock	2½ cups
juice of 1–2	lemons	juice of 1–2
freshly ground black pepper		
55g (2oz) each	celery, green or red (bell) pepper and cucumber, finely chopped	2oz each

Method

1 Put the tomatoes in a large pan with the garlic, onion, oil, wine and stock.
2 Bring to the boil and simmer for 1 hour.
3 Purée the soup in a food processor then put through a sieve to remove the pips.
4 Add lemon juice and pepper to taste, bearing in mind that flavours get dulled by chilling.
5 Chill the soup and, just before serving, add the chopped vegetables.

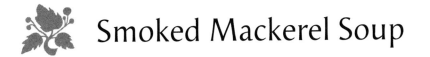

Smoked Mackerel Soup

Source of: calcium, vitamin D, potassium, EFAs
This is a very filling soup – a meal in itself. The smoked mackerel will give it lots of flavour so you should not need any seasoning.

Ingredients

SERVES 4

METRIC (IMPERIAL)		AMERICAN
170g (6oz)	onions, peeled and roughly sliced	1½ cups
285g (10oz)	floury potatoes, scrubbed and diced	2 cups
115g (4oz)	smoked mackerel fillets, skinned	4oz
1 litre (1¾ pints)	water	4¼ cups
140ml (5fl oz)	medium sherry	⅔ cup
4 tablespoons	plain live yoghurt	4 tablespoons

Method

1 Put the onions, potatoes and 85g (3oz) of the mackerel into a large saucepan with the water.
2 Bring to the boil and simmer gently for 15–20 minutes or until the potatoes are quite cooked.
3 Remove from the pan and purée in a food processor.
4 Return to the saucepan and add the rest of the smoked mackerel, broken into small pieces, and the sherry.
5 Reheat gently but do not boil.
6 Serve with a swirl of yoghurt in the middle of each dish.

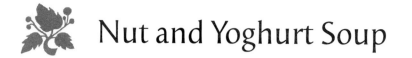

Nut and Yoghurt Soup

Source of: calcium, magnesium, potassium, EFAs
An unusual and delicious soup inspired by a Persian recipe in Claudia Roden's wonderful book, Middle Eastern Food. *You can serve it either hot or cold.*

Ingredients

Metric (Imperial)		American
2 tablespoons	sunflower or olive oil	2 tablespoons
2	onions, very finely chopped	2
¼ bulb	fennel, very finely chopped	¼ bulb
55g (2oz)	walnuts or pecans, coarsely chopped	½ cup
85g (3oz)	pine nuts	⅔ cup
1.5 litres (2½ pints)	hot water	6¼ cups
	sea salt and freshly ground black pepper	
400ml (14fl oz)	plain live yoghurt	1¾ cups

Method

1 Heat the oil in a large pan and fry the onions and fennel until they are a pale, golden colour.
2 Add the walnuts or pecans, 55g (2oz/½ cup) of the pine nuts and the water.
3 Season lightly with salt and pepper.
4 Bring to the boil and simmer, covered, for 15–20 minutes, then purée in a food processor.
5 Beat the yoghurt vigorously, add a ladleful of the hot soup and beat well. Gradually pour the mixture back into the soup, stirring all the while, then reheat very gently to just below boiling point.
6 Adjust the seasoning to taste and serve at once, sprinkled with the extra pine nuts.

Chilled Cucumber Soup
with Radish or Smoked Salmon

Source of: calcium, vitamins C and D, EFAs (salmon version)
A lovely, refreshing soup for a hot summer's day.

Ingredients

SERVES 4

METRIC (IMPERIAL)		AMERICAN
1 medium-sized	cucumber, roughly chopped	1 medium-sized
12 largish	spring onions (scallions), trimmed	12 largish
juice of 2	lemons	juice of 2
570ml (1 pint)	plain live yoghurt	2½cups
	sea salt	
	Tabasco	
10 large	radishes, grated	10 large
or		
4 small slices	smoked salmon, finely chopped	4 small slices

Method

1 Purée the unpeeled cucumbers with the spring onions (scallions) in a food processor.
2 Turn the mixture into a bowl and stir in the lemon juice and yoghurt.
3 Season to taste with sea salt and a little Tabasco.
4 Add the grated radishes or chopped salmon and chill thoroughly before serving.

Mrs Blencowe's Green Pea Soup with Spinach

Source of: calcium, magnesium, vitamin C, potassium, EFAs
A lovely deep-green soup adapted from a 17th-century recipe. Mrs Blencowe was the wife of a Member of Parliament.

Ingredients

SERVES 6

METRIC (IMPERIAL)		AMERICAN
3 tablespoons	sunflower or rapeseed oil	3 tablespoons
455g (1lb)	fresh or frozen green peas	3¼ cups
2 small	leeks, finely sliced	2 small
1	clove garlic, finely chopped	1
2	rashers green back bacon, cut into very small dice	2
1.2 litres (2 pints)	low-salt chicken or vegetable stock or water	5 cups
55g (2oz)	fresh or frozen (defrosted) leaf spinach	1 cup
55g (2oz)	white cabbage, very finely sliced	1 cup
1 stick	celery, de-stringed and finely chopped	1 stalk
½ small	lettuce, very finely chopped	½ small
large handful	parsley, finely chopped	large handful
1	carton mustard and cress	1
4 teaspoons fresh	chopped mint	4 teaspoons fresh or
2 teaspoons dried		2 teaspoons dried
	sea salt and freshly ground black pepper	
	pinch of mace	

Method

1 Heat a tablespoon of oil in a large pan and add the peas, leeks, garlic and bacon.
2 Fry gently until the vegetables are softened but not coloured.
3 Add the stock, bring to the boil and simmer for 20 minutes.
4 Liquidize or purée in a food processor.
5 Meanwhile, heat the rest of the oil in another pan and sweat the spinach, cabbage, celery, lettuce, parsley, mustard and cress and the mint until soft.
6 Add the puréed peas to the sweated mixture and mix well.
7 Season lightly with salt, pepper and mace before serving.

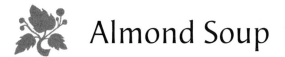

Almond Soup

Source of: calcium, magnesium, potassium, EFAs
This rich and unusual soup is based on a medieval recipe and works equally well hot or cold.

Ingredients

SERVES 4

METRIC (IMPERIAL)		AMERICAN
2	cloves	2
1	blade mace	1
1	bay leaf	1
55g (2oz)	ham, diced	¼ cup
2 sticks	celery, diced	2 stalks
1.2 litres (2 pints)	low-salt chicken stock or water	5 cups
200g (7oz)	ground almonds	2 cups
90ml (3fl oz)	medium sherry	⅓ cup
	white pepper	
4 tablespoons	creamy Greek yoghurt (optional)	4 tablespoons
	flaked almonds to decorate	

Method

1 Put the herbs and spices in a small muslin bag or infuser and place in a pan with the ham, celery and stock.
2 Bring to the boil and simmer for 30 minutes.
3 Add the almonds and simmer for another 15 minutes.
4 Remove the herb bag and purée the soup in a processor, then strain it through a coarse sieve.
5 Add the sherry and pepper. If necessary, you can also add a little sea salt although it should not need it.
6 Serve warm or chilled. If you wish, you can stir a tablespoon of creamy yoghurt into each bowl just before serving, although you may prefer to keep the simple flavour of the almonds. Sprinkle each bowl with a few flaked almonds.

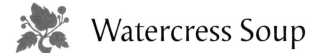

Watercress Soup

Source of: calcium, magnesium, vitamin C, potassium
The sea vegetables give this soup a delicious flavour without the need for any added salt.

Ingredients

METRIC (IMPERIAL)		AMERICAN
455g (1lb)	potatoes, scrubbed and sliced	3¼ cups
4	cloves garlic, peeled and sliced	4
200g (7oz)	watercress	7 cups
large handful	parsley	large handful
1.2 litres (2 pints)	water	5 cups
2 teaspoons	dried sea vegetables	2 teaspoons
285ml (½ pint)	coconut milk	1⅓ cups
handful	fresh mint, chopped	handful

Method

1 Put the potatoes, garlic, half the watercress and half the parsley into a large pan with the water and the sea vegetables.
2 Bring to the boil and simmer for 20–30 minutes or until the potatoes are quite cooked.
3 Purée the soup in a food processor.
4 Return to the pan, add the remains of the watercress and parsley, chopped finely, plus the coconut milk.
5 Serve the soup warm or cold, adding the freshly chopped mint just before serving.

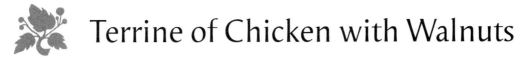

Terrine of Chicken with Walnuts

Source of: calcium, magnesium, potassium, EFAs
This lovely pâté can be used as a starter or with a salad for a light lunch. The walnuts turn slightly violet as they cook – which makes it look much more interesting!

Ingredients   SERVES 6

METRIC (IMPERIAL)		AMERICAN
1 small	chicken	1 small
570ml (1 pint)	water	2½ cups
255g (9oz)	piece of green bacon or gammon	9oz
55g (2oz)	broken walnuts or pecans	½ cup
10	peppercorns, lightly crushed	10
1 small	clove garlic, crushed	1 small
1 tablespoon	brandy	1 tablespoon

Method

1   Poach the chicken in the water for 30–40 minutes or until cooked.
2   Remove the chicken, cool it slightly, then take off the flesh and chop it into reasonably small pieces.
3   Reduce the stock by boiling it fast for about 10 minutes.
4   Boil the bacon in unsalted water for about 20 minutes or until cooked. Let it cool then cut it into dice.
5   Mix the chicken in a bowl with the bacon, walnuts, peppercorns, garlic and brandy. Add 90ml (3fl oz/⅓ cup) of the reduced stock and mix in well.
6   Heat the oven to 180°C/350°F/Gas Mark 4.
7   Grease a terrine dish and spoon in the mixture. Cover with baking foil.
8   Bake, in a *bain-marie*, for 75 minutes.
9   Remove the terrine from the oven, cool it slightly then weight it for at least 12 hours.
10 When it is absolutely cold, turn it out and slice to serve.

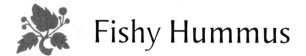

Fishy Hummus

Source of: calcium, vitamins C and D, EFAs
*For those who find it hard to eat their required amount of oily fish, this is an excellent way of
'disguising the medicine'.*

Ingredients

METRIC (IMPERIAL)		AMERICAN
2 x 115g (4oz) tins or	whole sardines or pilchards	2 x 4oz cans
170g (6oz)	smoked mackerel, smoked salmon or smoked trout	6oz
2 x 395g (14oz) tins	chickpeas (garbanzo beans), drained	2 x 14oz cans
3–4	cloves garlic, peeled	3–4
½ teaspoon	ground cumin	½ teaspoon
juice of 2	lemons	juice of 2
2 tablespoons	fresh parsley, finely chopped	2 tablespoons
	freshly ground black pepper	

Method

1   If you are using any of the smoked fish, skin them and remove any bones, if necessary.
2   Put the chickpeas (garbanzo beans), garlic, cumin, lemon juice and smoked fish or the sardines
    or pilchards, with their oil from the tin, in a food processor and purée until the mixture is as
    smooth as you want it. (Some like their purées quite coarse, while others prefer them very
    smooth.)
3   Add the parsley, pepper and extra lemon juice to taste.
4   Serve with pitta breads, toast, crudités or a salad.

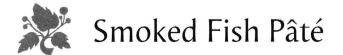

Smoked Fish Pâté

Source of: calcium, magnesium, vitamins C and D, EFAs
Another excellent way of boosting your intake of essential fatty acids. You can use the cheap off-cuts of
smoked salmon to be had in most supermarkets or smoked trout or smoked mackerel fillets.

Ingredients SERVES 6

METRIC (IMPERIAL)		AMERICAN
200g (7oz)	smoked mackerel, smoked trout or smoked salmon, skinned and boned, if necessary	7oz
55g (2oz)	sunflower spread	¼ cup
170g (6oz)	plain fromage frais	6oz
2 slices	wholemeal (wholewheat) brown bread freshly ground black pepper	2 slices
juice of	2–3 lemons	juice of

Method

1 Flake the fish into a mixing bowl with the spread and fromage frais.
2 Depending on how smooth you want the pâté, either beat them well with a wooden spoon or purée them in a food processor.
3 Crumble the slices of bread and beat into the pâté.
4 Season to taste with freshly ground black pepper and lemon juice.
5 Serve with toast, crackers, oatcakes or a salad.

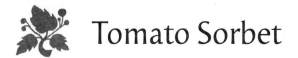

Tomato Sorbet

Source of: calcium, vitamin C, potassium
A lovely, fresh starter for a really hot day.

Ingredients   SERVES 6

METRIC (IMPERIAL)		AMERICAN
2 handfuls	parsley	2 handfuls
900g (2lb)	ripe tomatoes	2lb
1 teaspoon	Worcester sauce	1 teaspoon
115ml (4fl oz)	dry white wine	½ cup
	sea salt and freshly ground black pepper	

Method

1 Chop the parsley fairly finely in a food processor.
2 Remove most of the parsley from the processor and put in the tomatoes, with the Worcester sauce and white wine.
3 Purée them then rub the mixture through a strainer. You will get a rather pale pink and fluffy liquid.
4 Add the parsley and season to taste.
5 Pour into an ice-cream maker and churn-freeze.
6 If you do not have an ice-cream maker, put in a bowl and place in the freezer. Remove every 20 minutes while it is freezing and stir vigorously to prevent large ice crystals forming.
7 Remove from the freezer 15 minutes before serving to allow it to soften slightly.
8 Serve with crackers.

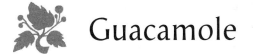

Guacamole

Source of: vitamin C, potassium
Although you can buy guacamole in most stores, the home-made variety still tastes MUCH better.

Ingredients

SERVES 6

METRIC (IMPERIAL)		AMERICAN
3	ripe avocados	3
1 small	onion, peeled and very finely chopped	1
1–2 (depending on taste)	cloves garlic, crushed	1–2 (depending on taste)
2	firm tomatoes, skinned, seeded and finely chopped	2
4–8	black olives, stoned and finely chopped	4–8
approx. 2 tablespoons	lemon juice	approx. 2 tablespoons
several drops	Tabasco	several drops

Method

1 Stone (pit) and peel the avocados.
2 If they are really ripe, you should be able to purée them with a wooden spoon in a bowl. If not, purée them in a food processor.
3 Add the onion and garlic and mix well.
4 Fold in the tomatoes and olives – how many of the latter will depend how keen you are on olives.
5 Season to taste with the lemon juice and Tabasco.
6 Serve the guacamole as a dip with crudités or as a pâté with hot brown toast.
7 Take care to cover the guacamole tightly if it is not to be used immediately as, like all avocado dishes, it will lose its colour if exposed to the air.

CHAPTER 14

Fish

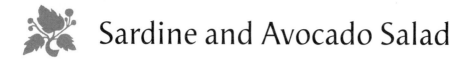

Sardine and Avocado Salad

Source of: calcium, vitamins C and D, potassium, EFAs
This is such an easy salad to make for one person for lunch that we have given the ingredients for a single portion. You can change the salad ingredients or just multiply them as you feel inclined! There should be enough flavour in the dressings for you not to need extra salt.

Ingredients

SERVES 1

METRIC (IMPERIAL)		AMERICAN
6	thin slices cucumber, halved or quartered	6
2	spring onions (scallions), trimmed and chopped	2
1 stick	celery or ¼ head fennel, finely sliced/chopped	1 stalk
½ small	green lettuce, chopped	½ small
½	avocado, peeled and chopped	½
handful	sprouted seeds	handful
small handful	parsley, chopped	small handful
1 tablespoon	mayonnaise	1 tablespoon
1 tablespoon	plain live yoghurt	1 tablespoon
1 tablespoon	olive oil	1 tablespoon
juice of ½	lemon	juice of ½
	freshly ground black pepper	
2	tinned sardines	2

Method

1 Mix all the vegetables gently together with the seeds and parsley.
2 In a separate bowl, mix the mayonnaise and yoghurt, olive oil, lemon juice and pepper.
3 Add to the vegetables and toss well.
4 Serve arranged on a plate with the two sardines.

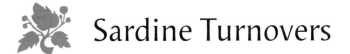

Sardine Turnovers

Source of: calcium, vitamins C & D, EFAs
These turnovers are good for lunch boxes, picnics or served with a salad.

Ingredients

METRIC (IMPERIAL)		AMERICAN
340g (12oz)	shortcrust pastry	12oz
approx. 12	anchovies, chopped	approx. 12
3 x 125g (4½oz) tins	sardines	3 x 4½oz cans
12	spring onions (scallions), trimmed and chopped	12
juice of 2 large	lemons	juice of 2 large

Method

1 Heat the oven to 180°C/350°F/Gas Mark 4.
2 Roll out the pastry and cut it into six circles, each 15–20cm (6–8 inches) in diameter.
3 Mix the chopped anchovies with the sardines (drained and roughly broken up), the spring onions (scallions) and the lemon juice.
4 Heap up one-sixth in the middle of each piece of pastry.
5 Fold the pastry over, damp the edges and pinch them together as for a Cornish pasty (meat turnover). You can either fold one side over the other and press them together on the working surface or you can bring both sides up and press them together on the top.
6 Carefully transfer the pasties, with a fish slice or metal spatula, onto a baking tray and bake for 15–20 minutes or until the pastry is cooked and lightly tanned.
7 Serve warm or cold.

Leek, Garlic and Cherry Tomato Marmalat with Tuna

Source of: vitamins C and D, potassium, EFAs
Fresh tuna steaks are now quite easy to find. If you cannot find (or do not like) tuna, you could use any other firm fish instead. A marmalat is a type of stew.

Ingredients

SERVES 4

METRIC (IMPERIAL)		AMERICAN
8 tablespoons	sunflower or olive oil	8 tablespoons
8 medium	leeks, trimmed and thickly sliced crossways	8 medium
12 large	cloves garlic, peeled but left whole	12 large
24	cherry tomatoes	24
2 heaped teaspoons	dried oregano	2 heaping teaspoons
4	fresh tuna steaks	4
	freshly ground black pepper	

Method

1 Put the oil in a heavy open pan with the leeks.
2 Cook gently for several minutes, then add the garlic cloves, tomatoes and oregano.
3 Stir well together and cook over a relatively brisk heat, stirring regularly for 10–15 minutes. The tomatoes will break down in the cooking to provide plenty of liquid.
4 Turn the heat down slightly and continue to cook gently for a further 10–15 minutes to allow the flavours to mature, but check regularly to make sure it is not drying out. If so, add a little white wine or water.
5 Meanwhile, lay the tuna steaks out on some aluminium foil, grind a little black pepper over each and dribble over a little oil.
6 Cook under a hot grill (broiler) for 4–5 minutes.
7 Turn, pepper, oil and cook for a further 4–5 minutes until done.
8 Serve on a bed of the marmalat with freshly steamed green beans.

Tuna Curry with Coconut Milk and Peanuts

Source of: calcium, magnesium, vitamins C and D, potassium, EFAs
If you do not like coriander (cilantro) leaves, substitute flat-leaved French parsley. The curry is best if you can use fresh tuna as the tinned variety will tend to disintegrate.

Ingredients

SERVES 6

METRIC (IMPERIAL)		AMERICAN
4 tablespoons	rapeseed or sunflower oil, if you are using fresh tuna	4 tablespoons
25g (1oz)	ginger root, peeled and finely sliced	1oz
6 large	cloves garlic, peeled and sliced	6 large
1 small	green chili pepper, seeded and finely sliced	1 small
2 medium	green (bell) peppers, seeded and sliced	2 medium
3 tablespoons	medium curry powder	3 tablespoons
565g (1¼ lb)	fresh tuna steaks or tuna steaks canned in oil	1¼ lb
395g (14oz)	cooked or canned chickpeas (garbanzo beans), drained	2⅓ cups
570ml (1 pint)	coconut milk	2½ cups
115g (4oz)	unsalted peanuts	⅘ cup
juice of 2–3	limes or lemons	juice of 2–3
2 handfuls	coriander (cilantro) leaves, chopped	2 handfuls

Method

1 Put the rapeseed or sunflower oil (or the oil from the cans of tuna) into a heavy, wide pan.
2 Add the ginger root, garlic, chili, green (bell) pepper and curry powder and cook together for 3–4 minutes.
3 If you are using fresh tuna, cut it into cubes and add it to the mixture, along with the chickpeas (garbanzo beans) and coconut milk.
4 Bring to the boil and simmer, covered, for 15 minutes.
5 If you are using canned tuna, add the chickpeas (garbanzo beans) and coconut milk and cook for 10 minutes, then add the tuna and continue to cook for a further 5 minutes.
6 Finally, add the peanuts and the lime or lemon juice to taste.
7 Serve the curry, liberally sprinkled with the fresh coriander (cilantro), with lots of freshly cooked rice and a green salad.

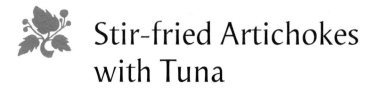

Stir-fried Artichokes with Tuna

Source of: calcium, magnesium, vitamins C and D, potassium, EFAs
A quick but tasty stir-fry which can be made with fresh or canned tuna.

Ingredients

SERVES 4

METRIC (IMPERIAL)		AMERICAN
3 tablespoons	sunflower oil	3 tablespoons
3	fresh green chili peppers, carefully seeded and finely sliced	3
3 large	cloves garlic, peeled and thinly sliced	3 large
6	spring onions (scallions), trimmed and chopped	6
285g (10oz)	fresh or canned tuna	10oz
170g (6oz)	fennel, trimmed and sliced	6oz
200g (7oz)	Jerusalem artichokes, scrubbed and cut into thin matchsticks	7oz
115g (4oz)	pak choi or other green Chinese cabbage, chopped	2 cups
55g (2oz)	sunflower seeds	½ cup
	soya sauce	
	fresh parsley, roughly chopped	

Method

1 Heat the oil in a wide pan or wok and cook the chili peppers, garlic and spring onions (scallions) until lightly coloured.

2 If you are using fresh tuna, cut it into cubes. If you are using canned, drain it and break it up.

3 Add the fresh tuna with the fennel and artichoke to the vegetables, stir well and continue to cook briskly for a couple of minutes. If you are using canned tuna, just add the artichoke and fennel.

4 If you are using canned tuna, add it now along with the pak choi and sunflower seeds. Cook, uncovered, for a minute or two.

5 Reduce the heat, cover the pan and cook gently or sweat for around 15 minutes or until the artichoke is just cooked but still crisp.

6 Season lightly with soya sauce, add the parsley and serve at once.

Dutch Herring and Beetroot Salad

Source of: calcium, vitamins C and D, potassium, EFAs
A very tasty and filling north-European dish – and a great way to eat those wonderfully healthy herrings!

Ingredients

METRIC (IMPERIAL)		AMERICAN
255g (9oz)	baby beetroot (red beet), scrubbed	9oz
255g (9oz)	new potatoes, scrubbed	9oz
4	rollmops or ready-pickled herrings	4
100ml (3½ fl oz)	plain live yoghurt	⅜ cup
large handful	chopped fresh parsley	large handful
juice of 1 large	lemon	juice of 1 large
	sea salt and freshly ground black pepper	

Method

1   Steam the beetroot (red beet) and potatoes in separate steamers until just cooked through.
2   Cut the beetroot (red beet) into matchsticks and slice the potatoes.
3   Unroll the rollmops, flatten them out and cut into thin matchsticks.
4   Mix the fish, beetroot (red beet) and potatoes in a bowl, then add the yoghurt and parsley and mix the whole lot together until the fish and vegetables are thoroughly coated in the yoghurt.
5   Add the lemon juice and season lightly with sea salt and freshly ground black pepper.
6   Serve with lots of fresh wholewheat, rye or pumpernickel bread.

Lemon Sole Stuffed with Seaweed

Source of: calcium, magnesium, vitamin C, potassium, EFAs
The seaweed not only gives a lovely flavour but is full of nutrients and saves having to use salt.

Ingredients

METRIC (IMPERIAL)		AMERICAN
4 tablespoons	rapeseed or sunflower oil	4 tablespoons
2 medium	leeks, finely sliced	2 medium
1 small head	fennel, very finely chopped	1 small head
1 handful	mixed dried seaweeds	1 handful
1 tablespoon	wild rice	1 tablespoon
450ml (¾ pint)	low-salt fish or vegetable stock	2 cups
3 tablespoons	basmati or jasmine rice	3 tablespoons
1	egg	1
juice of 1	lemon	juice of 1
4 large fillets	lemon sole, skinned	4 large fillets
285ml (½ pint)	white wine or low-salt fish stock	1⅓ cups
115g (4oz)	green beans, trimmed and halved	1⅓ cups
2	courgettes (zucchini), wiped and sliced	2
115g (4oz)	fresh spinach or chard, chopped	2 cups
	parsley, to decorate	

Method

1 Heat 2 tablespoons of oil in a deep pan and gently sweat one of the leeks and the fennel, covered, for 5–10 minutes or until starting to soften.
2 Add the seaweeds, the wild rice and 285ml (10fl oz/1⅓ cups) of stock.
3 Bring to the boil and cook for 10 minutes.
4 Add the white rice and continue to simmer until all the rice is cooked, adding the rest of the stock if the rice is drying up.
5 Remove from the heat and stir in the egg and lemon juice.
6 Place a tablespoon of the rice mixture in the middle of each fillet of fish and roll up.
7 Place the rolls in an ovenproof or microwave dish. Add 285ml (10fl oz/1⅓ cups) of white wine or fish stock and cover the dish.
8 Either bake in a moderate oven for 30 minutes or in a microwave on full power for 7–10 minutes, or until the fish is cooked. Keep warm.
9 Roll the rest of the rice into teaspoon-size balls and bake for 20 minutes in a moderate oven. Keep warm.
10 Meanwhile, in another pan, heat the remaining 2 tablespoons of oil and add the remaining leek.
11 Cook gently for 10 minutes, then add the green beans, courgettes (zucchini) and spinach.
12 Cover and cook gently for 10–15 minutes or until the vegetables are all cooked.
13 To serve, place the four sole rolls around the outside of a dish and pile the vegetables in the middle. Dot the rice balls around the dish, pour over the juices from both the fish and the vegetables, decorate with parsley and serve at once.

Smoked Salmon Tagliatelle

Source of: magnesium, vitamins C and D, potassium, EFAs
This recipe can be quite economical if you use the smoked salmon offcuts now available in most supermarkets.

Ingredients

METRIC (IMPERIAL)		AMERICAN
2 tablespoons	rapeseed or olive oil	2 tablespoons
2 large	red (bell) peppers, seeded and finely sliced	2 large
1 level teaspoon	dried oregano	1 level teaspoon
250ml (9fl oz)	dry white wine	1¼ cups
small handful	fresh chives, chopped	small handful
285ml (10fl oz)	single (half and half) cream	1⅓ cups
200g (7oz)	smoked salmon, cut into thin matchsticks	1 cup
55g (2oz)	pine nuts	½ cup
juice of 1	lemon	juice of 1
	freshly ground black pepper	
455g (1lb)	fresh tagliatelle	1lb

Method

1 Heat the oil in a wide pan and gently fry the sliced red (bell) peppers with the dried oregano for 15–20 minutes or until the peppers are quite soft.

2 Add the wine, increase the heat and cook fast for a further 5 minutes to reduce the wine.

3 Add the chives and the cream, mix thoroughly, then add the salmon and pine nuts and reheat gently – do not boil or the sauce will curdle.

4 Season to taste with lemon juice and pepper. Cover, set aside and keep just warm.

5 Cook the tagliatelle in plenty of lightly salted, fast-boiling water for 4–5 minutes or until just *al dente*. Drain and turn into a warmed serving dish.

6 Spoon over the salmon sauce and serve at once.

Braised Salmon Steaks with Flageolet Beans

Source of: calcium, magnesium, vitamins C and D, potassium, EFAs
A very simple but delicious way of serving salmon.

Ingredients
SERVES 4

METRIC (IMPERIAL)		AMERICAN
1 small	leek, thinly sliced	1 small
2	courgettes (zucchini), thickly sliced	2
200g (7oz)	chopped fresh or frozen spinach (if you use frozen spinach make sure it is well defrosted and drained)	7oz
1 x 395g (14oz) tin	flageolet beans, drained	1 x 14oz can
4	salmon steaks	4
1	lemon, sliced	1

Method

1 Mix the leek, courgettes (zucchini), spinach and beans in the bottom of wide, deep frying pan (skillet).
2 Lay the salmon steaks on the vegetables and top each steak with a slice of lemon.
3 Cover the pan and bring gently to a simmer.
4 Continue to simmer for 20 minutes or until the steaks are cooked through.
5 Serve at once with their bed of vegetables.

Rolled Salmon with Mangetout

Source of: vitamin D, EFAs
A rather grand dish based on an 18th-century English recipe.

Ingredients

METRIC (IMPERIAL)		AMERICAN
1 medium (2kg/4½lb)	salmon, boned and skinned but with the two sides still in 1 piece	1 medium (4½lb)
200g (7oz)	mussels, freshly cooked, frozen or tinned	7oz
1 large slice	wholemeal (wholewheat) bread, crumbed	1 large slice
6 large sprigs	parsley, chopped	6 large sprigs
	sea salt and freshly ground black pepper	
½	freshly grated nutmeg	½
½ teaspoon	ground mace	½ teaspoon
1 small head	fennel, chopped	1 small head
large bunch	parsley	large bunch
1	lemon, sliced	1
40g (1½oz)	butter	1½oz
40g (1½oz)	flour	1½oz
4 teaspoons	grated horseradish (not horseradish cream or sauce)	4 teaspoons
90ml (3fl oz)	medium sherry	⅓ cup
565g (1¼lb)	mangetout, trimmed	5 cups

Method

1 Lay the two sides of salmon out on the counter, insides facing upwards.

2 Arrange the mussels, breadcrumbs and parsley down the middle of each.

3 Season them fairly lightly with salt and pepper and the nutmeg and mace.

4 Roll both up carefully and wrap or tie them in a piece of muslin to prevent them falling apart. If you do not have any muslin, a new J-cloth does very well.

5 Put both rolls in a pan just big enough to hold them with the fennel, parsley and lemon. Cover with water.

6 Cover the pan and bring very slowly to the boil. Simmer for 5 minutes then turn off the heat. Leave the fish to continue cooking in the water for at least another hour.

7 Remove the rolls of fish carefully from the pan and set them aside. Strain the fish stock.

8 In a separate pan, melt the butter gently. Add the flour, stir around well then add the horseradish.

9 Slowly stirring all the time, add 400ml (14fl oz/1¾ cups) of the fish stock. Continue to cook until the sauce thickens.

10 Cook for a few more minutes then add the sherry and season to taste if it needs it.

11 Just before you are ready to serve, steam the mangetout for 4–5 minutes or until they are just starting to soften but still retain some crunch.

12 Carefully unwrap the fish and lay the rolls on a platter.

13 Arrange the mangetout around the fish and make a geometrical pattern with them over the fish.

14 Serve while still warm with the sauce handed separately.

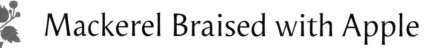

Mackerel Braised with Apple

Source of: vitamins C and D, EFAs
The apples and herbs counteract the richness of the mackerel, making this a very refreshing dish.

Ingredients

SERVES 4

METRIC (IMPERIAL)		AMERICAN
4 tablespoons	rapeseed or sunflower oil	4 tablespoons
2 large	onions, peeled and finely sliced	2 large
2 large	tart eating apples, peeled and sliced	2 large
1 large sprig	fresh rosemary or 2 teaspoons dried rosemary	1 large sprig
2 large or 4 small	mackerel, filleted or not, as you prefer	2 large or 4 small
200ml (7fl oz)	dry white wine	¾ cup
	sea salt and freshly ground black pepper	

Method

1 Heat the oil in a heavy pan, then add the onions, apples and rosemary.

2 Cover the pan and cook gently for 15 minutes or until the onions and apples are quite soft.

3 Lay the mackerel on top of the onion mixture, season lightly, pour around the wine, re-cover and continue to cook gently for a further 15–20 minutes or until the fish are cooked.

4 Serve at once with rice or potatoes and a green vegetable.

Parsnip and Smoked Mackerel Crumble

Source of: calcium, magnesium, vitamins C and D, potassium, EFAs
A really tasty, homely crumble.

Ingredients

METRIC (IMPERIAL)		AMERICAN
680g (1½lb)	parsnips, scrubbed and thinly sliced	5 cups
4 tablespoons	rapeseed or sunflower oil	4 tablespoons
340g (12oz)	tomatoes, sliced medium-thick	2 cups
225g (8oz)	button mushrooms, sliced	2½ cups
4	smoked mackerel fillets, skinned and flaked	4
140ml (5fl oz)	low-salt fish stock or water	⅔ cup
2 thick slices	wholewheat bread, crumbed	2 thick slices
85g (3oz)	grated Parmesan	1½ cups
1 tablespoon	sesame seeds	1 tablespoon
25g (1oz)	butter	1oz

Method

1 Heat the oven to 180°C/350°F/Gas Mark 4.
2 Steam the sliced parsnips for 10–15 minutes until nearly cooked.
3 Pour 2 tablespoons of oil into an ovenproof casserole and lay half the parsnip slices in the bottom, covered by half the sliced tomatoes.
4 Use the rest of the oil to briskly fry the mushrooms, then mix them with the flaked mackerel and lay this over the tomatoes.
5 Lay the rest of the parsnips over the fish mixture, and top with the remaining tomatoes.
6 Pour over the fish stock or water, cover then bake for 30–40 minutes.
7 Remove from the oven.
8 Mix the breadcrumbs with the Parmesan and sesame seeds and spread over the tomatoes.
9 Dot with the butter and brown under a grill (broiler) for a couple of minutes before serving with potatoes and a green vegetable.

CHAPTER 15

Meat and Poultry

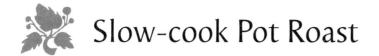

Slow-cook Pot Roast

Source of: calcium, magnesium, vitamin C, potassium, EFAs
If you cook this really slowly, the flavour will be quite delicious (you won't need any seasoning) and it will be wonderfully tender. The extra juice will make the most mouth-watering broth.

Ingredients

SERVES 6

METRIC (IMPERIAL)		AMERICAN
approx. 2kg (4½lb)	pot roast of beef	approx. 4½lb
6 small	onions, peeled and left whole	6 small
12	cloves garlic, peeled and left whole	12
6	button mushrooms	6
3 large	carrots, scrubbed and halved	3 large
4–6	bay leaves	4–6
20	black peppercorns	20
2 glasses	red wine	2 glasses
55g (2oz)	broken walnuts	½ cup

Method

1 Put the meat in a large, heavy, flame-proof lidded casserole which holds it fairly snugly.
2 Surround it with the onions, garlic, mushrooms and carrots, add the bay leaves, black peppercorns and the wine, then add water until the meat is covered.
3 Cover the casserole and cook in a low oven (150°C/300°F/Gas Mark 2) or over a very low heat for 4–6 hours. You could also cook it in a slow cooker overnight.
4 Allow the meat to cool in the juices, then chill until the fat solidifies.
5 Remove the fat, add the broken walnuts and gently reheat the casserole in a moderate oven (180°C/350°F/Gas Mark 4) for 45 minutes or until it is heated through. You could also reheat it in a microwave for 4–5 minutes on full power.
6 Serve with baked potatoes and a green vegetable.

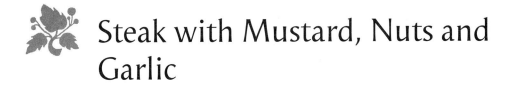

Steak with Mustard, Nuts and Garlic

Source of: calcium, magnesium, vitamin C, potassium, EFAs
The dressing gives the steaks a wonderful crunchy crust.

Ingredients

SERVES 4

METRIC (IMPERIAL)		AMERICAN
25g (1oz)	broken walnuts	¼ cup
25g (1oz)	hazelnuts	⅕ cup
4 large	cloves of garlic	4 large
6 heaped teaspoons	wholegrain mustard	6 heaping teaspoons
4	good rump, sirloin or fillet steaks	4

Method

1 Pulverize the walnuts and hazelnuts in a food processor but be careful not to process them for too long and turn them into paste.
2 Mash the garlic to a pulp with the point of a knife.
3 Mix the pulped garlic with the nuts and the mustard and generously coat both sides of each steak. Leave it aside for anything from half an hour to 2 hours.
4 To cook the steaks, place them under a very hot grill (broiler) for 2–8 minutes per side, depending on the thickness of the steak and how rare you like it. Take care not to put the steak too close to the grill (broiler) and burn the coating.
5 Turn the steaks halfway through cooking, scrape up any mustard dressing that may have fallen through the rack and spread it back on the steak.
6 Serve with a baked potato and a green salad.

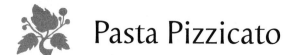

Pasta Pizzicato

Source of: vitamin C, potassium, EFAs
A lovely, spicy pasta dish – serve with a large, cool, green salad.

Ingredients

SERVES 4

METRIC (IMPERIAL)		AMERICAN
2 tablespoons	sunflower or chili oil	2 tablespoons
4	cloves garlic, peeled and sliced	4
2–4	red chili peppers, depending on how hot you want the sauce	2–4
2 sticks	celery, finely chopped	2 stalks
1 x 395g (14oz) tin	chopped tomatoes	1 x 14oz can
1 heaped tablespoon	tomato purée (paste)	1 heaping tablespoon
115g (4oz)	chorizo or other well-spiced sausage, diced	1 cup
	sea salt and black pepper (optional)	
340g (12oz)	dried pasta shapes (penne or shells)	4 cups

Method

1 Heat the oil in a heavy pan with the sliced garlic.
2 Remove the pith and seeds from the chili peppers, slice finely and add to the pan, along with the chopped celery.
3 Cover the pan and sweat over a low heat for 15 minutes.
4 Add the tomatoes, tomato purée (paste) and the sausage, re-cover the pan and continue to cook gently for 30 minutes until the flavours are well amalgamated and the sauce somewhat reduced.
5 Season to taste, if needs it.
6 Cook the pasta in plenty of fast-boiling, lightly salted water for 5–8 minutes or until just cooked.
7 Drain the pasta and mix in the sauce before serving – with a green salad to cool the heat!

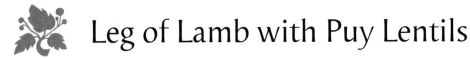

Leg of Lamb with Puy Lentils

Source of: calcium, potassium
*The full flavour of this dish comes out only if it is allowed to mature for at least 24 hours so, ideally,
cook it the day before you want to eat it.*

Ingredients

SERVES 6

METRIC (IMPERIAL)		AMERICAN
2 tablespoons	rapeseed or sunflower oil	2 tablespoons
6 tablespoons	puy lentils	6 tablespoons
3 medium	leeks, trimmed and halved	3
2–3	parsnips, halved lengthways and cut in rounds	2–3
10	button mushrooms, halved or quartered	10
395g (14oz)	baby potatoes, scrubbed	14oz
2 teaspoons each	dried marjoram and thyme	2 teaspoons each
2	bay leaves	2
½ teaspoon	ground coriander (cilantro)	½ teaspoon
1 teaspoon	black peppercorns	1 teaspoon
1 small	leg of lamb	1 small
6 cloves	garlic, peeled	6
200ml (7floz)	red wine	¾ cup
450ml (16fl oz)	low-salt vegetable or chicken stock	2 cups
	sea salt (optional)	

Method

1 Put the oil in the bottom of a heavy casserole with the lentils, leeks, parsnips, mushrooms, pota-toes, herbs and spices and mix well together.
2 Cut six slits in the lamb and insert the garlic cloves, then place it on top of the vegetable and lentil mixture.
3 Add the red wine and stock, bring slowly to the boil and simmer very gently for 2 hours. Alternatively, bake the casserole in a low oven (170°C/325°F/Gas Mark 3) for 2 hours.
4 Remove from the oven and set aside to cool overnight.
5 Before serving, reheat the casserole over a low heat or in a medium oven for 35–40 minutes.
6 Season to taste, if necessary, with sea salt and serve with lots of green vegetables and brown rice.

North-African Rolled Lamb

Source of: calcium, magnesium, vitamin C, potassium, EFAs
This dish, with its nuts and apricots, has quite a North-African feel to it. You can serve it either hot or cold, although you need to trim the fat really well if you are to serve it cold.

Ingredients

SERVES 6

METRIC (IMPERIAL)		AMERICAN
2kg (4½lb)	shoulder or leg of lamb	4½lb
1 teaspoon	coriander (cilantro) seeds	1 teaspoon
25g (1oz)	whole almonds	⅛ cup
25g (1oz)	pine nuts	⅛ cup
55g (2oz)	dried apricots, chopped	¼ cup
455g (1lb)	fresh spinach or defrosted frozen spinach leaf	8 cups
2 x 395g (14oz) tins	chickpeas (garbanzo beans), drained	2 x 14oz cans
	sea salt, freshly ground black pepper and ground nutmeg	
large sprig	fresh mint or 1 teaspoon dried mint	large sprig

Method

1 Bone the lamb or buy a boned joint (which should weigh approximately 1kg/2lb). Lay the boned shoulder or leg of lamb out on a counter.
2 Crush the coriander (cilantro) seeds lightly with a rolling pin then mix them with the nuts and apricots and spread over the lamb.
3 Roll the meat up and tie it neatly.
4 If you are using fresh spinach, wash it thoroughly then wilt it for 2–3 minutes in a large saucepan.
5 Mix the spinach with the chickpeas (garbanzo beans) and season lightly with salt, pepper and ground nutmeg.
6 Spoon into the bottom of an ovenproof casserole or saucepan just big enough to accommodate the lamb.
7 If you are using fresh mint, lay it over the vegetables, otherwise sprinkle them with the dried mint.
8 Lay the lamb over the top. Pour in a small wine glass of water. Cover the pan.
9 Either cook slowly over a low heat or in a moderate oven (180°C/350°F/Gas Mark 4) for 1 hour.
10 Remove the meat from the pan and cut the string.
11 Spoon the vegetable and pulse mixture onto a serving dish, lay the lamb on top and serve at once.

Duck with Orange and Apple Sauce, Pine nuts and Green Peppercorns

Source of: calcium, magnesium, potassium, EFAs
A much less rich and cloying version of the classic duck à l'orange.

Ingredients

METRIC (IMPERIAL)		AMERICAN
2kg (4½lb)	duck with giblets	4½lb
1 small	tart apple, peeled and chopped	1 small
1 teaspoon	green peppercorns	1 teaspoon
1 medium	onion, peeled and roughly chopped	1 medium
1 stick	celery, chopped	1 stalk
1	tomato, quartered	1
sprig	parsley	sprig
140ml (5fl oz)	red wine	⅔ cup
285ml (10fl oz)	water	1⅓ cups
2	oranges	2
15g (½oz)	butter	½oz
15g (½oz)	flour	½oz
55g (2oz)	pine nuts	½ cup
	sea salt	

Method

1. Heat the oven to 180°C/350°F/Gas Mark 4.
2. Prick the duck's skin thoroughly, fill its cavity with the apple and green peppercorns and roast on a rack in a roasting tin for approximately 1½ hours.
3. Meanwhile, put the giblets of the duck (reserving the liver), the onion, celery, tomato, parsley, wine and water into a large pan, bring to the boil and simmer for 45 minutes.
4. Carefully peel the rind off the oranges, removing as little pith as possible. Cut it into thin matchsticks and blanch it for a couple of minutes in boiling water.
5. Squeeze the juice from the oranges and set aside.
6. When the duck is cooked, remove it from the rack and pour off as much of the fat as you can, reserving the juices.
7. Melt the butter in a saucepan, add the duck liver chopped small and cook for a couple of minutes.
8. Add the flour, stir well and cook for another minute or two, then add the juices from the pan together with the apple (well mashed) and peppercorns from the middle of the duck.
9. Stir well again then gradually add 285ml (10fl oz/1⅓ cups) of the strained stock and the juice from the 2 oranges.

10. Stir all well together, bring to the boil and simmer for 5–10 minutes to allow the sauce to thicken.

11. Meanwhile, carve the duck and lay it in a warmed serving dish, removing as much or as little of the fatty (but crisp) skin as you want.

12. Strain the sauce, return it to the pan, add the orange rinds and pine nuts and reheat.

13. Season the sauce with a little sea salt if it needs it and pour over the duck.

14. Serve at once with green vegetables and really baby new potatoes, if they are available.

Chicken and Broccoli Risotto with Pistachios

Source of: calcium, magnesium, vitamin C, potassium, EFAs

Ingredients

SERVES 4

METRIC (IMPERIAL)		AMERICAN
4 tablespoons	rapeseed or sunflower oil	4 tablespoons
3 sticks	celery, chopped smallish	3 stalks
½ a large	green pepper, diced	½ a large
115g (4oz)	broccoli, the stalk chopped small and the heads chopped roughly	2 cups
1 medium	courgette (zucchini), diced	1 medium
6 heaped tablespoons	brown rice	6 heaping tablespoons
450ml (16fl oz)	water	2 cups
90ml (3fl oz)	dry white wine	⅓ cup
200g (7oz)	cooked chicken or turkey meat, diced	1 cup
25g (1oz)	pistachio nuts, halved	¼ cup
juice of 1	lemon	juice of 1
	sea salt and freshly ground black pepper	
generous handful	chopped parsley, chives or fresh coriander (cilantro)	generous handful

Method

1 Heat the oil in a heavy pan and add the celery, pepper and broccoli stalks. Cook gently until beginning to soften.

2 Add the courgette (zucchini), stir around for a minute or two, then add the rice. Again, stir for a minute or two then add the liquid.

3 Bring to the boil and simmer, uncovered, for 10 minutes or until the rice is just starting to soften.

4 Add the broccoli florets and the turkey or chicken meat.

5 Continue to cook until the liquid has almost evaporated and the rice is cooked, adding a little more water if necessary.

6 Add the pistachios and season to taste with lemon juice, sea salt, if necessary, and black pepper.

7 Serve warm or cold, generously sprinkled with the fresh herbs.

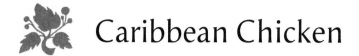

Caribbean Chicken

Source of: vitamin C, potassium, EFAs
A dashing and exotic dish – good for a steamy summer night.

Ingredients

Serves 4

Metric (Imperial)		American
3 tablespoons	sunflower or rapeseed oil	3 tablespoons
1 large	red (bell) pepper, seeded and sliced	1 large
200g (7oz)	okra (ladyfingers), topped, tailed and sliced thickly across	7oz
1 small	fresh or dried red chili pepper	1 small
395g (14oz)	boned raw chicken, breast or leg	14oz
455g (1lb)	tomatoes, roughly chopped	2½ cups
pinch	ground coriander (cilantro)	pinch
1 large	banana	1 large
	sea salt and freshly ground black pepper	

Method

1 Heat the oil in a pan and briskly fry the pepper and okra until both are softening.
2 Add the chili pepper and the cubed chicken and continue to fry briskly until the chicken is lightly browned all over.
3 Add the tomatoes and coriander (cilantro), cover the dish and cook over a very low heat for 25 minutes or until the chicken is cooked. If you cook it too quickly, the tomatoes will dry up and you will need to add a little water or white wine.
4 Once the chicken is cooked, add the banana (peeled and sliced thickly), cook for a couple of minutes, then adjust the seasoning to taste.
5 Serve hot with lots of brown rice and a really good green salad.

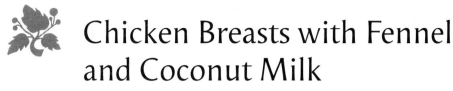

Chicken Breasts with Fennel and Coconut Milk

Source of: calcium, magnesium vitamin C, potassium
Another rather exotic chicken dish – although this one has hints of the Far East rather than the Caribbean.

Ingredients

SERVES 6

METRIC (IMPERIAL)		AMERICAN
6	chicken breasts	6
1 medium	onion, chopped	1 medium
1 wine glass	dry white wine	1 wine glass
1 tablespoon	sunflower or rapeseed oil	1 tablespoon
200g (7oz)	leeks, trimmed and very finely sliced	1¾ cups
1 bulb	fennel, trimmed and very finely sliced	1 bulb
200g (7oz)	fresh spinach or defrosted frozen leaf spinach	4 cups
25g (1oz)	potato flour	1oz
850ml (1½ pints)	coconut milk	3¾ cups
handful	fresh coriander (cilantro) leaves, chopped	handful
juice of 1–2	fresh limes	juice of 1–2
	sea salt and white pepper	

Method

1 Put the chicken breasts in a pan with the onion and the wine. Add water until the breasts are just covered.
2 Bring slowly to the boil and simmer gently for 30 minutes or until they are cooked. Take out and drain.
3 Meanwhile, heat the oil in a wide, heavy pan. Add the leeks and fennel, cover and sweat gently for 15–20 minutes, or until the vegetables are quite soft.
4 Add the chicken breasts with the spinach.
5 Mix the potato flour with a little of the coconut milk to make a smooth paste, then add to the pan, along with the rest of the coconut milk.
6 Cover the pan again and continue to cook gently for a further 10 minutes, until the sauce has thickened slightly.
7 Add the coriander (cilantro), the lime juice and salt and pepper to taste.
8 Serve at once with plenty of basmati rice and a salad or green vegetable such as mangetout.

Smoked Chicken with Avocado and Nectarine Salad

Source of: calcium, magnesium, vitamin C, potassium, EFAs
This is a delightful salad for a warm evening. The rich smoothness of the smoked chicken and avocado combined with the fresh tang of the nectarine and lime or lemon juice works particularly well. The amount of oak-smoked chicken may not seem a lot for four people, but it is quite rich and you can slice it much more thinly than a fresh chicken. You can use the salad as a starter (in which case there would be enough for six) or as a main course with a good green salad and some fresh brown bread.

Ingredients
SERVES 4

METRIC (IMPERIAL)		AMERICAN
½	oak-smoked chicken	½
	sea salt and freshly ground black pepper	
juice of approx. 1 small	lemon or lime	juice of approx. 1 small
approx. 3 tablespoons	walnut oil	approx. 3 tablespoons
1 large	ripe avocado	1 large
2	ripe nectarines	2
small bunch	fresh chives	small bunch

Method

1 Slice the chicken thinly and lay it out on a platter. If you have a big enough platter, you can lay the chicken round the outside and pile the salad in the middle.
2 Make a dressing with the salt, pepper, lemon or lime juice and oil.
3 Peel the avocado and slice it fairly thinly crossways.
4 Slice the nectarines into similar-sized pieces. Mix together gently with the avocado and dress them carefully so as not to bruise either fruit.
5 Pile the fruit in the centre of the serving dish or serve in a separate bowl.

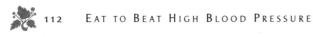

CHAPTER 16

Vegetables and Vegetarian Dishes

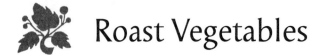

Roast Vegetables

Source of: calcium, vitamin C, potassium, EFAs
You can use almost any vegetable to create a dish of roast vegetables. This is a particularly delicious and attractive combination but feel free to experiment.

Ingredients

SERVES 6

METRIC (IMPERIAL)		AMERICAN
6–8 tablespoons	sunflower or rapeseed oil	6–8 tablespoons
3 small	sweet potatoes, peeled and cut into 3 fat rounds	3 small
1 bulb	celeriac, peeled and cut into large dice	1 bulb
2 medium	red (bell) peppers, seeded and quartered	2 medium
2 medium	yellow (bell) peppers, seeded and quartered	2 medium
12	cherry tomatoes	12
1 x 395g (14oz) tin	artichoke hearts, drained	1 x 14oz can
4	bay leaves	4
2–3 teaspoons	dried mixed herbs	2–3 teaspoons

Method

1 Heat the oven to 180°C/350°F/Gas Mark 4.
2 Put the oil in a wide, ovenproof dish with the sweet potatoes and the celeriac.
3 Cover with a lid or foil and cook for 40 minutes.
4 Remove from the oven and add the peppers, tomatoes, artichoke hearts and bay leaves.
5 Sprinkle over the mixed herbs and stir everything well to make sure all the ingredients are covered in oil.
6 Return to the oven, uncovered, for a further 45 minutes, stirring every now and then to make sure nothing burns.
7 Serve alone or as an accompaniment to a main dish.

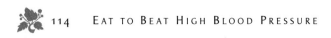

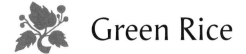

Green Rice

Source of: calcium, magnesium, vitamin C, potassium, EFAs
You can serve this dish as a vegetable or add two sliced avocados and a handful of walnuts or pecan nuts and serve it as a vegetarian main course.

Ingredients

SERVES 6

METRIC (IMPERIAL)		AMERICAN
2 tablespoons	sunflower or rapeseed oil	2 tablespoons
6	spring onions (scallions), trimmed and chopped	6
2	hot green chili peppers, seeded and thinly sliced	2
2 handfuls	fresh spinach leaves	2 handfuls
15	cardamom pods, bruised	15
340g (12oz)	white Patna or Chinese green rice	12oz
100ml (3½fl oz)	dry white wine	⅜ cup
approx. 570ml (1 pint)	water or low-salt vegetable stock	2½ cups
2 tablespoons	pine nuts	2 tablespoons
juice of ½–1	lemon	juice of ½–1
	sea salt and freshly ground black pepper	
large handful	fresh chopped coriander (cilantro) or parsley	large handful

Method

1 Heat the oil in a large, flat pan, add the spring onions (scallions), chili peppers and spinach leaves and cook gently for 4–5 minutes.
2 Add the cardamom pods and rice, stir well and continue to cook for a few minutes.
3 Add the wine and 500ml (18fl oz/2¼ cups) of the water or stock. Bring to the boil and simmer briskly until the rice is cooked, adding extra liquid as needed.
4 When the rice is done, add the pine nuts and then season to taste with the lemon juice and salt and pepper.
5 Add the coriander (cilantro) or parsley and serve at room temperature.

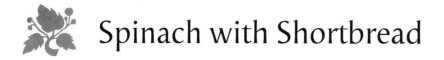

Spinach with Shortbread

Source of: calcium, magnesium, vitamin C, potassium

Ingredients

Metric (Imperial)		American
40g (1½oz)	melted butter	1½oz
55g (2oz)	plain (all purpose) flour	½ cup
25g (1oz)	well-flavoured cheese, grated	¼ cup
1.5kg (3½lb)	fresh spinach, well washed, thoroughly drained and with any heavy stalks removed	3½lb
1 handful	dried seaweed – arame or a mixed sea vegetable	1 handful
1 tablespoon	sunflower oil	1 tablespoon
25g (1oz)	plain (all purpose) flour	⅕ cup
285ml (10fl oz)	low-salt vegetable stock	1⅓ cups

Method

1 Heat the oven to 180°C/350°F/Gas Mark 4.
2 Mix the melted butter into the first measure of flour, add the cheese and mix to a soft dough.
3 Roll out on a well-floured board, cut into hearts or other biscuit shapes and bake for 10 minutes. Set aside.
4 Briefly cook the spinach with the seaweed in 5cm (2 inches) of boiling water, drain thoroughly and chop, squeezing out as much of the remaining water as you can.
5 Heat the oil in a large, wide pan, add the second measure of flour and cook for a couple of minutes.
5 Add the spinach and continue to cook for 5 minutes.
6 Then add the stock and cook for a further couple of minutes to warm the sauce through. Season to taste if it needs it.
7 Turn the spinach onto a heated serving dish and decorate with the shortbread biscuits before serving.

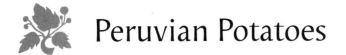

Peruvian Potatoes

Source of: calcium, magnesium, potassium, EFAs
In South America, the potato is, quite rightly, valued as a food in its own right – not just as an accompaniment to other foods. The dish is best eaten when the potatoes are still just warm, but if you want to prepare it ahead of time and eat it cold, it is still excellent.

Ingredients   SERVES 4

METRIC (IMPERIAL)		AMERICAN
395g (14oz)	new potatoes, scrubbed	14oz
3 tablespoons	walnut or sunflower oil	3 tablespoons
1 small	onion, thickly sliced	1 small
2	cloves garlic, finely chopped	2
3 small	green chili peppers, seeded and finely chopped (if using dried chilies you will need to soak them in boiling water first)	3 small
55g (2oz)	broken walnuts or pecans	½ cup
55g (2oz)	crumbly white cheese	½ cup
200g (7oz)	cooked shrimps or prawns	2 cups
250ml (9floz)	semi-skimmed milk	1¼ cups
	sea salt	

Method

1   Steam or microwave the potatoes until cooked, then halve them lengthways.
2   Meanwhile, heat the oil and gently fry the onion and garlic over a low heat until the onion is golden.
3   Put the oil, onions, garlic, chili peppers, walnuts or pecans, cheese and 115g (4oz/1 cup) of the shrimps or prawns in a food processor and purée, gradually adding the milk to reduce the consistency to a thick sauce. Add extra milk if it seems too thick.
4   Season lightly to taste with sea salt.
5   While the potatoes are still warm, lay them out on a serving dish, pour over the sauce and decorate with the remaining shrimps or prawns.

Jersey Royals with Asparagus and Pistachio Nuts

Source of: calcium, magnesium, potassium, EFAs
This is a really delicious way to serve potatoes for a lunch or a light supper dish followed by a salad.
Jersey Royals are particularly delicious but any young new potatoes will do.

Ingredients

SERVES 4

METRIC (IMPERIAL)		AMERICAN
900g (2lb)	Jersey Royal or other new potatoes, lightly scrubbed	2lb
565g (1¼lb)	thick asparagus spears, trimmed	1¼lb
2 tablespoons	virgin sunflower oil or olive oil	2 tablespoons
115g (4oz)	pistachio nuts, shelled and roughly chopped	1 cup
	or 50g (2oz) ready-shelled pistachios, chopped	
	sea salt and freshly ground black pepper	
juice of ½–1	lemon	juice of ½–1

Method

1 Steam the potatoes for 10–15 minutes or until cooked.
2 Halve any that are too big and spread out over the base of a serving dish.
3 Meanwhile, in a separate pan or steamer, steam the asparagus for 8–10 minutes or until just cooked.
4 Arrange the asparagus spears over the potatoes in the dish.
5 Heat the oil and lightly fry the chopped pistachio nuts in it for a couple of minutes.
6 Pour over the potatoes and asparagus.
7 Lightly season with sea salt and freshly ground black pepper and squeeze over the lemon juice.
8 Serve at once.

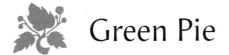

Green Pie

Source of: calcium, magnesium, vitamin C, potassium
An unusual quiche. If you can get fresh herbs rather than dried, it makes the quiche taste deliciously fresh.

Ingredients

SERVES 6

METRIC (IMPERIAL)		AMERICAN
115g (4oz)	wholemeal (wholewheat) flour	⅘ cup
115g (4oz)	plain (all purpose) white flour	⅘ cup
115g (4oz)	butter or low-fat spread	½ cup
a little	water	a little
170g (6oz)	broccoli florets, broken up quite small and steamed for 6 minutes or until half-cooked	3 cups
2 tablespoons	pumpkin seeds	2 tablespoons
25g (1oz)	pistachio nuts, shelled and halved	¼ cup
115g (4oz)	fresh chard, chopped	4oz
handful	chopped parsley	handful
handful	mixed fresh herbs – rosemary, basil, marjoram or whatever else you can get or	handful
1 heaped teaspoon	mixed dried herbs	1 heaping teaspoon
4	eggs	4
450ml (16fl oz)	low-salt vegetable stock freshly ground black pepper	2 cups

Method

1 Heat the oven to 180°C/350°F/Gas Mark 4.
2 Mix the flours together and rub in the butter or spread until you have a sandy consistency.
3 Add enough water to make a stiff paste and roll out.
4 Line a 20-cm (8-inch) flan dish with two-thirds of the pastry, weight it with some aluminium baking foil and some beans and bake it for 20 minutes.
5 Meanwhile, put the broccoli in a large bowl with the pumpkin seeds and the pistachio nuts. Chop the chard and parsley and add it along with the herbs.
6 In a separate bowl, beat 3 of the eggs, add the stock and season lightly. Add the liquid mixture to the green mixture and mix well.
7 If you want to cover the pie with a pastry lid, put a pie support in the middle of the dish then pour in the mixture.
8 Cover the pie with the remaining pastry and paint the lid with the remaining egg, beaten.
9 Bake for 45 minutes with no lid and 55 minutes with a lid. Serve warm or cold.

Mushroom and Sunflower Seed Flan

Source of: calcium, magnesium, vitamin C, EFAs
A tasty flan based on an 18th-century recipe.

Ingredients

METRIC (IMPERIAL)		AMERICAN
85g (3oz)	butter or low-fat spread	1/3 cup
170g (6oz)	wholemeal (wholewheat) flour	1 heaping cup
3 tablespoons	sunflower oil	3 tablespoons
225g (8oz)	mushrooms, whole if they are button, halved or quartered if they are open	2 cups
85g (3oz)	fresh rocket or spinach, chopped fairly small	1½ cups
170g (6oz)	palm hearts (tinned), cut in two or three pieces depending on size	6oz
2 heaped tablespoons	sunflower seeds	2 heaping tablespoons
	sea salt and freshly ground black pepper	
juice of ½–1	lemon	juice of ½–1

Method

1 Heat the oven to180°C/350°F/Gas Mark 4.
2 Make the pastry by rubbing the butter into the flour then adding enough water to make a firm dough.
3 Roll the pastry out and line a 25-cm (10-inch) flan dish. Prick the bottom, line it with aluminium baking foil, weight it with beans or rice and bake for 15 minutes with the foil in, then 10 minutes without, to get it nice and crisp.
4 Meanwhile, heat the oil in a heavy pan and add the mushrooms. Fry briskly for several minutes.
5 Add the chopped rocket or spinach, stir well, cover the pan and cook for a further couple of minutes.
6 Remove the lid and add the palm hearts and sunflower seeds and continue to cook for a few minutes to warm the palm hearts through.
7 Season lightly with sea salt, pepper and lemon juice.
8 Spoon into the flan case, spread out over the bottom and serve at once.

Broccoli au Gratin with Butter Beans

Source of: calcium, magnesium, vitamin C, potassium, EFAs
A filling and tasty variation on traditional cauliflower cheese.

Ingredients

SERVES 6

METRIC (IMPERIAL)		AMERICAN
170g (6oz)	onions, roughly chopped	1⅓ cups
680g (1½lb)	broccoli florets	12 cups
55g (2oz)	sunflower spread	¼ cup
55g (2oz)	flour	½ cup
1 tablespoon	wholegrain mustard	1 tablespoon
570ml (1 pint)	semi-skimmed milk or low-salt vegetable stock	2½ cups
140g (5oz)	well-flavoured hard cheese	1 heaping cup
55g (2oz)	Parmesan	1 cup
	freshly ground black pepper to taste	
1 x 395g (14oz) tin	butter beans, drained	1 x 14oz can
25g (1oz)	flaked almonds	⅓ cup
25g (1oz)	fresh brown breadcrumbs	½ cup

Method

1 Steam or microwave the onions and broccoli florets until just cooked but still slightly *al dente*. Set aside.
2 Meanwhile, melt the spread in the pan and add the flour to make a roux. Add the mustard then gradually add the milk or stock, stirring continuously until you get a smooth sauce.
3 Add most of the hard cheese (leaving a little for the topping) and the Parmesan and stir until melted.
4 Season with black pepper – the cheese should make it salty enough.
5 Carefully stir in the broccoli, butter beans and almonds and, mixing carefully, gradually bring back to just below boiling point. Turn into a flame-proof serving dish.
6 Mix the remaining cheese with the breadcrumbs and sprinkle over the top of the dish.
7 Pass the dish under the grill (broiler) for a couple of minutes to lightly brown the top. Serve at once.

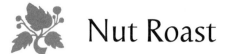

Nut Roast

Source of: calcium, magnesium, potassium, EFAs
This traditional vegetarian dish tastes great hot or cold.

Ingredients

METRIC (IMPERIAL)		AMERICAN
1 tablespoon	sunflower or rapeseed oil	1 tablespoon
1 medium	onion, peeled and finely chopped	1 medium
2 large	cloves garlic, peeled and finely chopped	2 large
2 heaped teaspoons	dried mixed herbs	2 heaping teaspoons
200g (7oz)	mixed nuts – whatever combination you fancy	7oz
200g (7oz)	brown breadcrumbs or cooked brown rice	7oz
2 medium	eggs, beaten	2
	sea salt, freshly ground black pepper	
	and nutmeg	

Method

1 Heat the oven to 180°C/350°F/Gas Mark 4.
2 Heat the oil and add the onions, garlic and mixed herbs. Fry gently for 5–8 minutes or until the onion has softened.
3 Put the nuts into a food processor and process until they are as crushed as you want. If you leave pieces too large, the loaf will tend to fall apart, but too finely ground and your loaf will not have much texture.
4 Add the nuts to the onions, along with the breadcrumbs or rice and the eggs.
5 Season lightly with a little sea salt, freshly ground pepper and nutmeg.
6 Line a 455g (1lb) loaf tin with oiled, greaseproof (wax) paper and spoon in the loaf. Pat down and flatten the top.
7 Bake for 30 minutes.
8 Serve hot or cold with vegetables or salad and with a little chutney or redcurrant jelly.

Flageolet Bean Salad with Artichoke Hearts

Source of: calcium, magnesium, vitamin D (with sardines), vitamin C, potassium, EFAs (with sardines)
A very pleasant, simple salad. If you want to make it more substantial (and up its EFA content), serve it with a couple of sardines for each person and wholemeal (wholewheat) toast.

Ingredients   SERVES 4

METRIC (IMPERIAL)		AMERICAN
4 tablespoons	olive oil	4 tablespoons
4 small	courgettes (zucchini), wiped, topped and tailed and thickly sliced	4 small
1 x 395g (14oz) tin	flageolet beans	1 x 14oz can
2 x 395g (14oz) tins	artichoke hearts	2 x 14oz cans
3 tablespoons	pumpkin seeds	3 tablespoons
200g (7oz)	fresh spinach, washed, well dried and chopped	4 cups
2 large handfuls	fresh parsley or coriander (cilantro), roughly chopped	2 large handfuls
juice of 1	lemon	juice of 1
	seaweed seasoning or a little sea salt	
	freshly ground black pepper	
8	fresh or tinned sardines (optional)	8

Method

1 Heat 2 tablespoons of the oil and briskly fry the courgettes (zucchini) until nicely browned and nearly soft.
2 Drain the beans and drain and quarter the artichoke hearts.
3 Mix the artichokes with the courgettes (zucchini) in a large salad bowl, then add the flageolets, pumpkin seeds, spinach and parsley or coriander (cilantro).
4 Mix well together, dress with the remaining oil and lemon juice and season to taste.
5 If you are using them, arrange the sardines on top of the salad before serving.

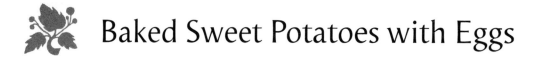

Baked Sweet Potatoes with Eggs

Source of: calcium, vitamin C, EFAs
You can serve this dish either as a vegetable (without the eggs) or as a supper or lunch dish (with the eggs). The sweet potatoes give it the most wonderful golden colour.

Ingredients

METRIC (IMPERIAL)		AMERICAN
900g (2lb)	sweet potatoes, peeled and sliced/diced	6½ cups
3–4 large	cloves garlic, peeled	3–4 large
1 tablespoon	pumpkin or walnut oil (if you find them difficult to get, sunflower or olive oil will be fine but not as tasty)	1 tablespoon
1 tablespoon	maple syrup or honey	1 tablespoon
2 tablespoons	sunflower seeds, roughly chopped	2 tablespoons
6	eggs	6

Method

1 Heat the oven to 180°C/350°F/Gas Mark 4.

2 Steam the sweet potatoes and garlic cloves for 15–20 minutes or until both are quite soft.

3 Purée in a food processor along with the oil and maple syrup or honey. (If you use the pumpkin oil you probably won't need any salt – if you use any of the others you may need to taste the purée and add a little salt.)

4 If you want to serve the purée as a vegetable, add the sunflower seeds, reheat and serve.

5 If you want to serve it as a main dish, spoon the purée into an ovenproof casserole and make six indentations in the mixture. Break an egg into each then sprinkle the sunflower seeds over the eggs.

6 Bake for 15–20 minutes or until the eggs are just set. Serve at once with a green salad or vegetable.

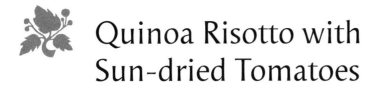

Quinoa Risotto with Sun-dried Tomatoes

Source of: calcium, vitamin C, potassium, EFAs
This dish requires access to a good health-food or fine-food store. Arame is a wonderful Japanese sea-weed; quinoa is a delicious, rice-like South American grain.

Ingredients   SERVES 6

METRIC (IMPERIAL)		AMERICAN
2 tablespoons	sunflower oil	2 tablespoons
4	fresh chili peppers (whatever 'heat' you like), seeded and sliced	4
handful	dried arame	handful
170g (6oz)	sun-dried tomatoes in oil, halved or quartered	6oz
9 tablespoons	quinoa grain	9 tablespoons
1 litre (1¾ pints)	low-salt vegetable stock	4½ cups

Method

1 Heat the oil in a pan and gently fry the sliced chilies for a few minutes.
2 Add the arame, tomatoes, quinoa and stock. Stir well.
3 Bring to the boil and simmer, uncovered, for 20–25 minutes or until the quinoa is cooked (it should still have some texture) and the liquid is largely absorbed. The dish should not need any further seasoning.
4 Serve alone with a salad or as an accompaniment to a main dish.

 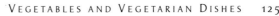

Buckwheat Pasta with Savoy Cabbage

Source of: calcium, magnesium, vitamin C, potassium, EFAs
A simple but surprisingly successful dish. If you wish to make it more substantial, add 115g (4oz/½ cup)
chopped ham to the finished dish.

Ingredients

SERVES 4

METRIC (IMPERIAL)		AMERICAN
4 tablespoons	sunflower oil	4 tablespoons
2	Spanish onions, roughly chopped	2
455g (1lb)	savoy cabbage, roughly chopped	8 cups
1 teaspoon	caraway seeds	1 teaspoon
230ml (8fl oz)	low-salt vegetable stock	1 cup
	sea salt and freshly ground black pepper	
255g (9oz)	buckwheat pasta in whatever shape you fancy	9oz

Method

1 Heat the oil in a large pan and gently fry the onions until just soft and lightly tanned.
2 Add the cabbage and continue to cook for a few minutes, then add the caraway seeds, stock and a little seasoning.
3 Simmer for 5–10 minutes or until the cabbage is cooked but still slightly crunchy.
4 Meanwhile, cook the pasta in fast-boiling water until just *al dente*.
5 Drain and mix into the cabbage.
6 If you are using the ham, add it to the dish and mix well.
7 Adjust seasoning to taste and serve at once.

Wild Mushroom and Hemp Pasta

Source of: vitamin C, EFAs
The dark, nutty taste of hemp pasta or soba noodles goes really well with the flavour of the mushrooms.

Ingredients

SERVES 4

METRIC (IMPERIAL)		AMERICAN
8 tablespoons	olive oil	8 tablespoons
4 tablespoons	walnut oil	4 tablespoons
1 large	leek, finely sliced	1 large
4 large	garlic cloves, peeled and finely sliced	4 large
15–20	cardamom pods, bruised	15–20
285g (10oz) each	shitake, oyster and portabellini mushrooms or	3 cups each
900g (2lb)	any combination of mushrooms you prefer, wiped and roughly sliced	10½ cups
455g (1lb)	dried hemp tagliatelle or Japanese soba noodles freshly ground black pepper	1lb
juice of 2	lemons	juice of 2
8	spring onions (scallions), trimmed and chopped small	8
large handful	fresh coriander (cilantro), chopped	large handful
200g (7oz)	soft but tangy goat, sheep or buffalo cheese	7oz

Method

1 Heat the oils in a wide, heavy pan and add the leek, garlic and cardamom pods.
2 Cook gently for 10 minutes or until the vegetables are quite soft.
3 Add the mushrooms and increase the heat. Cook briskly for 3–5 minutes or until the mushrooms are soft.
4 Meanwhile, cook the pasta in plenty of lightly salted fast-boiling water – the length of time will depend on the pasta you are using. When just *al dente*, drain and set aside.
5 Season the mushroom mixture with pepper and plenty of lemon juice.
6 Mix the mushrooms into the pasta, along with the spring onions (scallions) and sprinkle generously with fresh coriander (cilantro) or parsley.
7 Put a spoonful of cheese on top of each serving and allow to melt into the hot pasta.
8 Serve immediately.

CHAPTER 17

Desserts

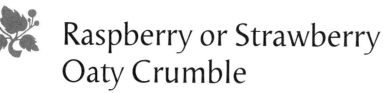

Raspberry or Strawberry Oaty Crumble

Source of: magnesium and vitamin C
A new concept in crumbles! If you want it to taste even fruitier, substitute pear and apple concentrate for the honey.

Ingredients

SERVES 4–6

METRIC (IMPERIAL)		AMERICAN
170g (6oz)	porridge oats	2 cups
55g (2oz)	wholemeal (wholewheat) flour	½ cup
85g (3oz)	butter or low-fat spread	⅓cup
2 tablespoons	good honey (or pear and apple concentrate)	2 tablespoons
565g (1¼lb)	fresh raspberries or strawberries	5 cups raspberries, 4 cups strawberries
2 heaped teaspoons	arrowroot	2 heaping teaspoons

Method

1 Heat the oven to 180°C/350°F/Gas Mark 4.
2 To make the crumble mixture, mix the oats and flour and rub in the butter. Mix in the honey or pear and apple concentrate.
3 Purée half of the raspberries or strawberries and chop the rest fairly roughly.
4 Put the arrowroot in a small pan and add a little of the purée. Stir until smooth, then add the rest of the purée.
5 Heat gently until the sauce thickens, then amalgamate it with the chopped raspberries or strawberries.
6 Spread half the crumble mixture over the bottom of a shallow baking dish or flan dish – at least 1-cm (½-inch) thick.
7 Spread the fruit mixture over the crumble and the rest of the crumble over the top.
8 Bake the crumble for 30 minutes.
9 Serve warm or cold – alone or with yoghurt, cream or ice cream.

Kiwi and Banana Pudding

Source of: calcium, magnesium, vitamin C, potassium, EFAs
A lovely, filling dessert for a winter's evening, with the added benefit of having no added sugar.

Ingredients

SERVES 6

METRIC (IMPERIAL)		AMERICAN
1 large Bramley cooking apple		2 large tart dessert apples
4	kiwi fruit, peeled and sliced	4
2–3	bananas, depending on size, peeled and sliced	2–3
3 tablespoons	fresh or frozen cranberries	3 tablespoons
2	eggs	2
2 tablespoons	plain (all purpose) flour	2 tablespoons
2 tablespoons	ground almonds	2 tablespoons
200ml (7fl oz)	soya or coconut milk	¾ cup

Method

1 Heat the oven to 180°C/350°F/Gas Mark 4.
2 Scrub the apple (apples), core, leave the skin on and chop very small.
3 Cook in 2 tablespoons water, covered, for 5–10 minutes, or until quite puréed. (If you are using dessert apples which do not pulp so easily, you may need to purée the apple in a food processor.)
4 Tip the apple into a pie dish and smooth over the bottom.
5 Lay the kiwi slices over the apple, and the banana over the kiwi. Sprinkle with the cranberries.
6 In a bowl, beat the eggs with the flour, almonds and milk and pour over the top of the fruit.
7 Bake, uncovered, for 50 minutes or until the custard is set and slightly browned.
8 Serve warm alone or with cream, yoghurt or ice cream.

Apple and Banana Crumble

Source of: magnesium, vitamin C, potassium, EFAs
The crisp crumble topping contrasts well with the soft fruit below.

Ingredients

METRIC (IMPERIAL)		AMERICAN
2 large	unpeeled cooking (tart dessert) apples, cored and chopped small	2 large
2 large	bananas, sliced	2 large
4 tablespoons	water	4 tablespoons
55g (2oz)	butter or low-fat spread	¼ cup
2 heaped tablespoons	honey or apple and pear concentrate	2 heaping tablespoons
115g (4oz)	porridge oats	1⅓ cups
25g (1oz)	wholemeal (wholewheat) flour	⅕ cup
25g (1oz)	sunflower seeds	¼ cup

Method

1 Preheat the oven to 180°C/350°F/Gas Mark 4.
2 Cook the apples and bananas together with the water, either on the hob or in a microwave until soft.
3 Dissolve the butter or spread with the honey or apple and pear concentrate in a pan or microwave
4 Stir in the oats, flour and sunflower seeds and mix well.
5 When the apples and bananas are cooked, transfer them to a pie dish, then spread the crumble over the top.
6 Cook for approximately 20 minutes or until the crumble has become golden brown.
7 Serve warm or at room temperature, alone or with low-fat yoghurt.

Strasbourg Nut and Apple Tart

Source of: calcium, magnesium, vitamin C, potassium, EFAs
A rather rich but delicious apple meringue tart.

Ingredients

SERVES 6

METRIC (IMPERIAL)		AMERICAN
200g (7oz)	plain (all purpose), sifted flour	1½ cups
pinch	baking powder	pinch
3	eggs	3
30ml (1fl oz)	water	⅛ cup
115g (4oz)	very soft butter or low-fat spread	½ cup
455g (1lb)	cooking (tart dessert) apples, peeled and chopped	4 cups
1 heaped tablespoon	dark molasses sugar	1 heaping tablespoon
60ml (2fl oz)	water	¼ cup
55g (2oz)	chopped walnuts or pecans	½ cup
1 tablespoon	sour cream	1 tablespoon
1 tablespoon	light molasses sugar	1 tablespoon
25g (1oz)	chopped or sliced almonds	¼ cup
15g (½oz)	plain (all purpose) flour	½oz

Method

1 Heat the oven to 180°C/350°F/Gas Mark 4.
2 Put a little of the flour in a bowl with the baking powder, 1 egg, the water and the butter or spread and mix thoroughly.
3 Gradually add the rest of the flour, always mixing in the same direction, until the paste coalesces into a ball.
4 Chill for 30 minutes, then roll out and line a 20-cm (8-inch) flan case.
5 Prick the bottom, line it with foil, weight it with beans and cook for 25 minutes.
6 Remove and lower the temperature to 150°C/300°F/Gas Mark 2.
7 Meanwhile, cook the apples with the dark molasses sugar and water until quite soft; mix them thoroughly with a fork then add the walnuts or pecans and sour cream.
8 Once the flan case is cooked, spoon the apple mixture into the bottom.
9 To make the topping, mix the remaining egg yolks with the light molasses sugar, chopped almonds and flour.
10 Whisk the whites, fold them into the mixture and spoon it over the apple.
11 Bake, uncovered, for one hour.
12 Take out and cool. The tart can be served warm or cold, by itself or with whipped cream, crème fraîche or yoghurt.

Chocolate and Orange Curd Tart

Source of: magnesium, vitamin C, potassium
The chocolate pastry gives an unusual flavour to this traditional citrus curd tart.

Ingredients

SERVES 6

METRIC (IMPERIAL)		AMERICAN
115g (4oz)	plain (all purpose) flour	1 scant cup
25g (1oz)	dark molasses sugar	1oz
25g (1oz)	cocoa powder	¼ cup
85g (3oz)	butter or low-fat spread	⅓ cup
Filling:		
55g (2oz)	butter	¼ cup
25g (1oz)	light molasses sugar	1oz
3	eggs	3
2	grated rind and juice of 2 large oranges	2
1	grated rind and juice of 1	1

Method

1　Heat the oven to 180°C/350°F/Gas Mark 4.
2　Mix together the flour, dark molasses sugar and cocoa powder. Cut and rub in the butter or spread and mix it to a firm dough with a little cold water.
3　Roll out the pastry and line a 20-cm (8-inch) flan case, reserving any bits of pastry left over.
4　Line the flan case with aluminium baking foil and weight with beans. Bake it blind for 20 minutes. Take care not to overcook it as its colour is too dark for you to be able to see when it is burning.
5　Reduce the oven temperature to 170°C/325°F/Gas Mark 3.
6　Meanwhile, make the filling by melting the butter in the top of a double boiler, or very gently in a heavy-bottomed pan.
7　Add the sugar then beat in the eggs, followed by the rind and juice of the oranges and lemon.
8　Cook the mixture over a low heat, stirring continually until the curd thickens. Take care not to boil or the mixture will curdle.
9　Spoon the filling into the flan case.
10　Roll out the remaining bits of pastry very thinly, cut into lattice strips and decorate the top of the flan.
11　Bake for a further 20 minutes to cook the lattice work.
12　Serve warm or cold, alone or with cream or yoghurt.

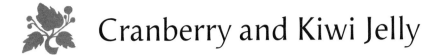

Cranberry and Kiwi Jelly

Source of: vitamin C
This makes quite a tart jelly as it has no added sugar, although both the liqueur and the cranberry juice contain sugar.

Ingredients

SERVES 4

METRIC (IMPERIAL)		AMERICAN
115g (4oz)	fresh or frozen cranberries	4oz
60ml (2fl oz)	cherry brandy (optional)	¼ cup
230ml (8fl oz)	cranberry juice	1 cup
or 285ml (10fl oz)	if you do not use the cherry brandy	1⅓ cups
20g (¾ oz)	gelatine	¾ oz
3	kiwi fruits	3

Method

1 Put the cranberries in a pan with the juice and cherry brandy, bring to the boil and simmer for 5 minutes or until the cranberries are soft. Remove the cranberries with a slotted spoon and set aside.

2 Sprinkle the gelatine over the hot liquid and allow it to melt completely.

3 Pour a very thin layer of the jelly into the bottom of a decorated jelly mould and allow to set.

4 Peel and slice 2 of the kiwis thinly.

5 Arrange some kiwi slices and some cranberries on the set jelly in a pattern. Cover with a little more jelly and allow to set again.

6 Continue this pattern until you have used up all the fruit and juice.

7 Put the mould in the refrigerator to set.

8 To serve, dip the container fairly briefly into a bowl of boiling water to loosen the edges (how long it takes will depend on the thickness and material of your jelly mould) then turn it onto a decorative plate, if you have one.

8 Slice the remaining kiwi fruit and arrange around the jelly.

10 Serve the jelly alone or with cream or yoghurt.

Lemon Sponge with Apricots

Source of: magnesium, vitamin C, potassium (dried apricots), EFAs
This lovely fresh-tasting sponge cake works equally well with fresh or dried apricots.

Ingredients

SERVES 6

METRIC (IMPERIAL)		AMERICAN
15	soft dried apricots or10 stoned fresh apricots, in season	15
4 tablespoons	brandy	4 tablespoons
5	eggs	5
170g (6oz)	light molasses sugar	1 scant cup
	rind and juice of 1 large lemon	
170g (6 oz)	plain (all purpose) flour	1 heaping cup
1 teaspoon	toasted sesame seeds	1 teaspoon

Method

1   Chop the apricots fairly small and soak them for up to 24 hours in the brandy. They should absorb most of it.
2   Heat the oven to 180°C/350°F/Gas Mark 4.
3   In an electric mixer, beat the eggs with the sugar until very light, fluffy and creamy.
4   Gently fold in the lemon rind, flour and lemon juice.
5   Line a 20-cm (8-inch) cake tin with greased greaseproof (wax) paper and pour in the cake mix.
6   Bake for 30 minutes or until a skewer comes out clean. Cool slightly in the tin then turn out onto a rack.
7   When entirely cold, cut the cake in half horizontally. Spread the brandy-soaked apricots over the cake and top it with the other half.
8   Sprinkle with extra lemon zest and sesame seeds to decorate.
9   Serve with cream, yoghurt or ice cream.

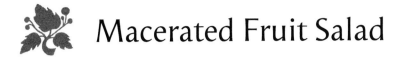

Macerated Fruit Salad

Source of: calcium, magnesium, vitamin C, potassium, EFAs
This traditional Middle Eastern way of serving fruit is very easy to prepare and quite delicious.

Ingredients

SERVES 6

METRIC (IMPERIAL)		AMERICAN
340g (12oz)	mixed dried fruits – choose from dates, prunes, apricots, raisins, figs	12oz
85g (3oz)	nuts – you can use pine nuts, flaked almonds or walnuts (pecans) or a mixture of 2	3oz
1 tablespoon	orange flower water	1 tablespoon

Method

1 Put the fruits, nuts and orange flower water into a bowl.
2 Just cover with cold water (filtered if possible).
3 Cover the bowl and set aside in a cool larder or the top shelf of the fridge for at least 36, preferably 48, hours. The fruits will melt into the water, creating a delicious syrup.
4 Serve at room temperature with cream or ice cream.

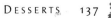

Apricot Nutmeg Ice Cream

Source of: calcium, magnesium, vitamin C, potassium, EFAs
An unusual, spicy ice cream with a distinctly Indian flavour.

Ingredients

METRIC (IMPERIAL)		AMERICAN
500ml (18fl oz)	semi-skimmed cow's or sheep's milk	2¼ cups
200ml (7fl oz)	coconut milk	¾ cup
1 level teaspoon	ground cinnamon	1 teaspoon
½–1 teaspoon	ground nutmeg (freshly ground if possible)	½–1 teaspoon
115g (4oz)	dried apricots	½ cup
2 level tablespoons	light molasses sugar	2 level tablespoons
25g (1oz)	toasted flaked or sliced almonds	⅓ cup

Method

1 Pour the milks into a pan with the spices and the apricots.
2 Bring slowly to the boil, simmer for a few minutes then cool completely.
3 When quite cold, purée in a food processor (how smooth you make it will depend on how 'bitty' you like your ice cream).
4 Add the sugar and the almonds and turn into an ice-cream maker to churn-freeze.
5 As with all ice creams, remove from the freezer to the fridge half an hour before you want to serve it.

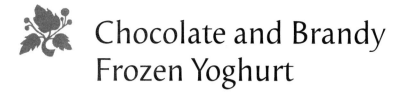

Chocolate and Brandy Frozen Yoghurt

Source of: calcium, magnesium, potassium
A real luxury ice cream – which still contains 'good' nutrients!

Ingredients

SERVES 4

METRIC (IMPERIAL)		AMERICAN
395g (14oz)	Greek-style yoghurt	14oz
170g (6oz)	good-quality bitter chocolate	1 cup
4 tablespoons	brandy	4 tablespoons
25g (1oz)	dark molasses sugar	1oz

Method

1 Beat the yoghurt until smooth with a wooden spoon or in a mixer.
2 Melt 115g (4oz/⅔ cup) of the chocolate over hot water or in a microwave.
3 Mix a little of the yoghurt into the chocolate, then stir the melted chocolate, brandy and sugar into the rest of the yoghurt.
4 Grate or chop the remaining chocolate and stir into the ice cream.
5 Put the mixture into an ice-cream maker and churn-freeze.
6 If you do not have an ice-cream maker, turn the mixture into a bowl and freeze until the edges are frozen and the centre stiff. Remove from the freezer and whisk hard with an electric or hand whisk. Replace the mixture in the freezer and leave to refreeze. Whisk twice more before the mixture is quite frozen to break down the ice crystals.
7 Serve directly from the ice-cream maker once it is just frozen stiff.
8 If it has been stored in the freezer, remove to the fridge 20–30 minutes before serving to allow the mixture to soften slightly.

CHAPTER 18

Baking

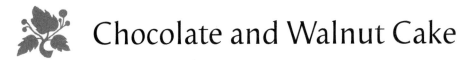

Chocolate and Walnut Cake

Source of: calcium, magnesium, potassium and EFAs
This lovely, moist, rich – but not over-sweet – cake can be eaten just as a cake or split, filled with icing
and topped with whole strawberries for a spectacular gateau.

Ingredients

METRIC (IMPERIAL)		AMERICAN
140g (5oz)	walnuts, ground in a food processor	1¼ cups
200g (7oz)	sunflower spread	1 scant cup
170g (6oz)	dark molasses sugar	1 scant cup
200g (7oz)	dark chocolate	1 heaping cup
6	eggs	6
140g (5oz)	self-raising flour	1 cup
Icing:		
200g (7oz)	dark chocolate	1 heaping cup
200g (7oz)	sunflower spread	1 scant cup
1 heaped teaspoon	instant coffee	1 heaping teaspoon

Method

1   Heat the oven to 180°C/350°F/Gas Mark 4 and line a 20-cm/8-inch cake tin with greased grease-proof (wax) paper.
2   Grind the walnuts in a food processor but take care not to leave them too long or they will turn into walnut paste.
3   Beat the sunflower spread with the sugar until light and fluffy.
4   Melt the chocolate in a microwave or a double boiler and beat into the sugar and spread.
5   Break the eggs and mix them in, each accompanied by a spoonful of flour.
6   Fold in the rest of the flour and the walnuts and spoon into the prepared cake tin.
7   Bake for 30–40 minutes or until a skewer comes out clean. Cool for a few minutes then turn onto a rack.
8   To make the icing, melt the chocolate in a microwave or double boiler.
9   Beat the spread until soft then beat in the chocolate.
10 Dissolve the coffee in 60ml (2fl oz/¼ cup) boiling water and beat into the icing.
11 Allow to cool until almost set then use to fill and cover the cake.

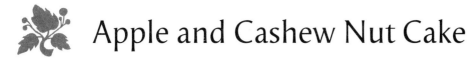

Apple and Cashew Nut Cake

Source of: calcium, magnesium, vitamin C, potassium
This nice, fruity sponge cake does not include any added sugar.

Ingredients

METRIC (IMPERIAL)		AMERICAN
140g (5oz)	butter or low-fat spread	⅔ cup
55g (2oz)	softened dried dates	½ cup
200g (7oz)	fresh dessert apples, grated (peel them if you want the texture to be really smooth, otherwise leave them unpeeled)	7oz
115g (4oz)	broken cashew nuts	1 scant cup
2 medium	eggs	2
115g (4oz)	wholemeal (wholewheat) flour, sifted with 2 level teaspoons baking powder	1 scant cup
juice of 1 small	orange	1

Method

1 Heat the oven to 180°C/350°F/Gas Mark 4.
2 In a food processor, combine the butter or spread with the dates and apples. When they are really well amalgamated, transfer to a bowl.
3 Grind the cashew nuts in a food processor until they are as fine as possible without turning into paste then mix them into the butter and apple.
4 Add the eggs, one at a time, with a tablespoon of flour with each.
5 Fold in the rest of the flour sifted with the baking powder, and the orange juice.
6 Transfer to a well-oiled round or square cake tin (lined with greaseproof/wax paper unless you are absolutely sure it will not stick) and bake for 45–50 minutes or until a skewer comes out clean.
7 Turn out onto a rack to cool.

Coffee and Walnut
or Pecan Sponge

Source of: calcium, magnesium, potassium, EFAs
This cake tastes excellent with its large pieces of walnut or pecan – and keeps very well in a tightly fitting tin or covered with clingfilm (plastic wrap).

Ingredients

METRIC (IMPERIAL)		AMERICAN
225g (8oz)	butter	1 cup
170g (6oz)	dark muscovado sugar	1 scant cup
3 medium	eggs	3 medium
285g (10oz)	white or wholemeal (all purpose or wholewheat) flour	2 cups
2 level teaspoons	baking powder	2 level teaspoons
1 level teaspoon	ground nutmeg	1 level teaspoon
1 level teaspoon	ground cinnamon	1 level teaspoon
small pinch	salt	small pinch
340ml (12fl oz)	strong black coffee	1½ cups
170g (6oz)	walnuts or pecans, roughly chopped, plus a few whole walnuts for decoration	1⅓ cups
200g (7oz)	dark chocolate	1 heaping cup

Method

1 Heat the oven to 180°C/350°F/Gas Mark 4.

2 Beat 170g (6oz/¾ cup) of the butter with the sugar until fairly light and fluffy.

3 Separate the eggs and beat the 3 egg yolks into the mixture.

4 Sift the flour with the baking powder, spices and salt.

5 Fold the flour into the butter and sugar mixture alternately with 285ml (10fl oz/1⅓ cups) of the coffee.

6 Stir in the chopped walnuts or pecans.

7 Whisk the egg whites until they hold their shape but are not stiff or dry, and mix and fold them carefully into the cake mixture.

8 Spoon into a 20-cm (8-inch) round cake tin – or a similar-capacity loaf tin – with a loose bottom or lined with greaseproof paper.

9 Bake for 50–60 minutes or until a skewer comes out clean.

10 Remove from the oven and the tin and cool on a rack.

11 To make the icing, beat the remaining butter until really soft.

12 Melt the chocolate over boiling water or in a microwave.

13 Heat the remaining coffee.

14 Gradually beat the butter and the hot coffee into the melted chocolate and, when thoroughly mixed, spread over the cake.

15 Arrange the whole walnuts on top and allow the icing to cool and harden before cutting.

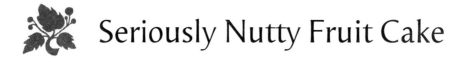

Seriously Nutty Fruit Cake

Source of: calcium, magnesium, vitamin C, potassium, EFAs
Not only is this cake high in all the nutrients you should be eating, it has no added sugar and tastes delicious. It makes a small but very rich cake and works really well as a Christmas cake.

Ingredients

Metric (Imperial)		American
115g (4oz)	butter or low-fat spread	½ cup
2 medium	ripe bananas	2 medium
rind and juice of 2	lemons	rind and juice of 2
2	eggs	2
85g (3oz) each	raisins and sultanas	½ cup each
170g (6oz)	soft dried apricots, roughly chopped	1 scant cup
25g (1oz) each	flaked (sliced) almonds and pine nuts	1oz each
55g (2oz)	broken walnuts or pecans	½ cup
55g (2oz)	toasted hazelnuts, roughly chopped	½ cup
85g (3oz)	rolled oats, lightly pulverized in a food processor	1 cup
85g (3oz)	plain white (all purpose) flour	½ cup
2 heaped teaspoons	baking powder	2 heaping teaspoons
2 teaspoons	ground nutmeg	2 teaspoons
1 teaspoon each	ground ginger and ground cinnamon	1 teaspoon each
2 tablespoons	brandy or orange/apple juice	2 tablespoons

Method

1 Heat the oven to 170°C/325°F/Gas Mark 3.
2 Purée the butter or low-fat spread with the banana and lemon rind and juice in a food processor. Lightly beat in the eggs.
3 Turn into a bowl and stir in the fruits and nuts, followed by the flours, baking powder, spices and, finally, the brandy or fruit juice. Make sure it is well mixed.
4 Line a 15-cm (6-inch) cake tin with greased greaseproof (wax) paper and spoon in the mixture. Smooth out and bake for 1 hour or until a skewer comes out clean.
5 Cool slightly in the tin then turn out and leave to get completely cold before cutting.

Oat-based Molasses Gingerbread

Source of: magnesium, potassium
A deliciously dark and sticky gingerbread.

Ingredients

METRIC (IMPERIAL)		AMERICAN
115g (4oz)	butter or low-fat spread	½ cup
115g (4oz)	dark molasses sugar	½ cup
225g (8oz)	black treacle	⅔ cup
4	eggs	4
225g (8oz)	rolled or porridge oats, powdered in a food processor	2½ cups
1 heaped teaspoon	baking powder	1 heaping teaspoon
2 heaped teaspoons	ground ginger	2 heaping teaspoons
1 heaped teaspoon	mixed spice	1 heaping teaspoon
1 heaped teaspoon	ground cinnamon	1 heaping teaspoon

Method

1 Heat the oven to 170°C/325°F/Gas Mark 3.
2 Melt the butter or spread, sugar and treacle together in a pan or microwave. Remove from the heat.
3 Beat the eggs into the melted mixture followed by the oats, baking powder and spices.
4 Pour into a greased loaf tin or cake tin and bake for 45 minutes or until a skewer comes out clean.
5 Take out of the oven and the tin and cool on a rack.

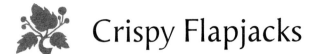

Crispy Flapjacks

Source of: calcium, magnesium, potassium, EFAs
This recipe makes rather delicious crispy flapjacks, which are less gooey than usual.

Ingredients

Metric (Imperial)		American
115g (4oz)	butter or low-fat spread	½ cup
55g (2oz)	dark molasses sugar	⅓ cup
55g (2oz)	golden syrup	⅙ cup
225g (8oz)	porridge oats	2½ cups
25g (1oz)	pine nuts	⅙ cup
25g (1oz)	sunflower seeds	¼ cup

Method

1. Heat the oven to 180°C/350°F/Gas Mark 4.
2. Dissolve the fat, sugar and syrup in a pan or microwave but do not let them boil or the flapjacks will go tacky rather than crisp.
3. Stir in the oats, nuts and seeds and mix together well.
4. With your fingers, press the mixture out in a thin layer in the bottom of a metal or Pyrex flan dish.
5. Cook the flapjack mixture for 30 minutes.
6. As soon as it is cooked, cut it into sections and cool slightly.
7. Remove the flapjacks from the tin and allow to cool on a rack.

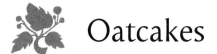

Oatcakes

Source of: magnesium
Delicious with cheese, pâté or just by themselves with soup or a salad. Also excellent for cocktail canapés.

Ingredients

METRIC (IMPERIAL)		AMERICAN
225g (8oz)	mixed oatmeals: fine, medium and pinhead	1⅓ cups
115g (4oz)	wholemeal (wholewheat) flour	1 scant cup
small pinch	salt	small pinch
1 level teaspoon	baking powder	1 level teaspoon
85g (3oz)	butter or low-fat spread	⅓ cup

Method

1 Heat the oven to 180°C/350°F/Gas Mark 4.

2 Put the oatmeal in a basin and sift in the flour, salt and baking powder.

3 Rub the fat in as for pastry and mix to a stiff dough with cold water.

4 Turn the mixture onto a board sprinkled with oatmeal.

5 Knead the dough lightly, roll it out thinly and cut into rounds with a glass or pastry cutter. Make the oatcakes whatever size you want.

6 Place them on a tray and bake for 20–25 minutes, keeping an eye on them to make sure they do not burn.

7 Cool on a rack and store in an airtight container or the freezer.

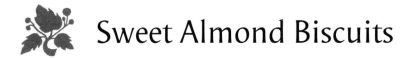

Sweet Almond Biscuits

Source of: calcium, magnesium, potassium, EFAs
Delicious little biscuits to serve with coffee or a dessert.

Ingredients

MAKES APPROX. 20 SMALL BISCUITS

METRIC (IMPERIAL)		AMERICAN
115g (4oz)	ground almonds	1⅓ cups
85g (3oz)	rice flour	½ cup
85g (3oz)	pale muscovado sugar	½ cup
25g (1oz)	butter or low-fat spread	1oz
2	egg whites	2

Method

1 Heat the oven to 180°C/350°F/Gas Mark 4.

2 Mix the almonds, rice flour and 55g (2oz/⅓ cup) of the sugar together.

3 Rub in the butter or spread followed by the egg whites.

4 With your hands, form the mixture into small balls and roll in the remaining sugar.

5 Place on a lightly oiled baking tray and press flat with a fork.

6 Bake for 15–20 minutes or until the biscuits are just turning golden.

7 Remove to a wire rack and allow to cool.

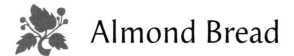

Almond Bread

Source of: calcium, magnesium, vitamin C, potassium, EFAs
This loaf is a cross between bread and a cake – but is very enjoyable and full of good nutrients.

Ingredients

METRIC (IMPERIAL)		AMERICAN
115g (4oz)	ground almonds	1⅓ cups
55g (2oz)	wholemeal (wholewheat) flour	½ cup
1 level teaspoon	baking powder	1 level teaspoon
55g (2oz)	dark molasses sugar	⅓ cup
25g (1oz)	melted butter	1oz
2	eggs, separated	2
juice and rind of 1	small lemon	juice and rind of 1

Method

1 Heat the oven to 180°C/350°F/Gas Mark 4.
2 Mix the almonds, flour, baking powder and brown sugar in a bowl.
3 Melt the butter and add it along with the egg yolks.
4 Beat the mixture well, then add the lemon rind and juice.
5 Whisk the egg whites until they hold their shape in soft peaks and mix them into the bread.
6 Pour the mixture into a 15-cm (6-inch) well-greased loaf tin.
7 Bake for 25 minutes or until the loaf has risen slightly and a skewer comes out clean.
8 Cool on a wire rack. The bread can be eaten alone or with butter.

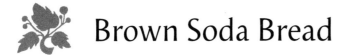

Brown Soda Bread

Source of: calcium, magnesium

A traditional Irish brown loaf – full of flavour and texture. It is said that the bread should be left for 24 hours before it is cut, but I have yet to meet a person who can resist the smell of it when warm... If you cannot get buttermilk, use plain live yoghurt (preferably sheep or goat) soured with the juice of half a lemon.

Ingredients

METRIC (IMPERIAL)		AMERICAN
565g (1¼lb)	coarse brown (wholewheat) flour	4 cups
140g (5oz)	strong white flour	1 cup
pinch	salt	pinch
1 tablespoon	bicarbonate of soda (baking soda)	1 tablespoon
570–850ml (1–1½ pints)	buttermilk	2½–3¾ cups

Method

1 Heat the oven to 190°C/375°F/Gas Mark 5.

2 Mix the dry ingredients thoroughly together.

3 Make a well in the middle and lightly mix in enough buttermilk to make a soft dough.

4 Shape the loaf into a round cob shape on a floured baking tin and cut a cross in the top.

5 Bake for 35–45 minutes or until the bottom sounds hollow when you tap it. It is a good idea to turn the loaf upside down for the last 10 minutes to make sure the bottom gets crisp.

6 Cool on a rack.

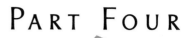

PART FOUR

Taking it Further

CHAPTER 19

High Blood Pressure
and Food Supplements

A number of food and herbal supplements are helpful for someone with high blood pressure. Those covered elsewhere in this book include olive oil (*Chapter 4*), omega-3 fish oils (*Chapter 5*), folic acid (*Chapter 6*), isoflavones (*Chapter 8*), garlic (*Chapter 9*) and green tea (*Chapter 10*). Those discussed in this chapter include:

* antioxidants
* calcium
* magnesium
* co-enzyme Q10
* hawthorn
* dandelion
* ginkgo
* padma 28
* lecithin and choline
* L-carnitine
* flaxseed oil
* hemp seed oil
* bilberry
* royal jelly
* specialist herbal medicines.

Food supplements are effective in helping to maintain a healthy circulation. If you want to take supplements, but are unsure where to start or worried about taking too much, I have developed my own range, Trilogy. This uses a simple, three-step process that helps make taking supplements as easy as one, two, three ...

Step 1: Select a vitamin and mineral formula based on your age (under or over 50).

Step 2: Add in an essential fatty acid formula (evening primrose or omega-3 fish oil based).

Step 3: Plus a specific nutrient formula (Healthy Heart & Circulation, Healthy Back & Joints, Healthy Resistance or Healthy Energy) if you have a particular health need.

For those with high blood pressure, a good basic regime would be to take:

🌺 Step 01: The enhanced vitamin and mineral supplement 50+, which supplies additional antioxidants and isoflavones.

🌺 Step 02: Omega-3 essential fatty acid formula, which supplies fish and extra virgin olive oil plus co-enzyme Q10 and extra vitamin E.

🌺 Step 03: Healthy Heart & Circulation, which supplies alpha-lipoic acid, garlic (allicin yield 1,500mcg), grapeseed, green tea and bilberry extracts.

For more information, visit www.trilogy.gb.com

Antioxidants

Antioxidants are protective substances that help to neutralize damaging oxidation reactions in the body. Most oxidations are triggered by free radicals – unstable molecular fragments that carry a negative electrical charge in the form of a spare electron. Free radicals try to lose this charge by colliding with other molecules and cell structures in an attempt to either pass on the spare electron, or to pinch a positive charge with which to neutralize it. This chemical process is known as oxidation, and one of the best-known examples is when iron oxidizes to form rust.

We need a certain amount of free-radical activity in the body but too much can trigger harmful chain reactions in which spare electrical charges are shunted from one chemical to another, damaging proteins, fats, cell membranes and genetic material. Oxidation of LDL-cholesterol in the circulation is necessary before scavenger cells will recognize the fat as harmful. The scavenger cells then try to remove the oxidized fat by engulfing it, quickly becoming overburdened and forming bloated 'foam' cells. These leave the circulation by squeezing between cells lining the artery wall where they become trapped and accumulate as part of the hardening and furring-up process. Lack of antioxidants, rather than excessive dietary fat intake, is now thought by many researchers to be the main underlying cause of atherosclerosis.

Free radicals are generated in a number of ways, including:

🌺 normal metabolic reactions
🌺 burning excess body fat while losing weight
🌺 exposure to environmental pollutants, x-rays or UVA sunlight
🌺 when exercising, during energy-production processes
🌺 smoking cigarettes
🌺 drinking alcohol
🌺 inhaling exhaust fumes
🌺 when taking certain drugs, especially antibiotics or paracetamol.

Smokers and people with diabetes generate more free radicals than usual.

You cannot avoid generating a certain number of free radicals, but you can minimize the amount of damage they do by ensuring your intake of antioxidants is high. Antioxidants are our main defence against free-radical attack. They work by quickly mopping up and neutralizing negative charges on free radicals before they can trigger a chain reaction. Several essential vitamins and minerals act as antioxidants. Of these, the most important are vitamins A, C and E and selenium. Other antioxidants are also available in supplement form, such as pine bark extracts, co-enzyme Q10, carotenoids (such as betacarotene, lutein and lycopene), plus bilberry, ginkgo, green tea or grapeseed extracts.

A scientific review of over 150 clinical trials published in the *Journal of the American Medical Association* showed that low intakes of many vitamins is a risk factor for heart disease, stroke and other major chronic health problems. In an accompanying paper, the authors actually state that *'Pending strong evidence of effectiveness from randomized trials, it appears prudent for all adults to take vitamin supplements.'* For those who find this difficult to believe, the reference is: 'Vitamins for Chronic Disease Prevention in Adults. Clinical applications'. Fletcher, R.H., Fairfield, K.M., *JAMA* 2002;287:3127–3129.

BENEFITS OF VITAMIN C

Vitamin C is an important antioxidant that protects fluid parts of the body from harmful oxidations. Lack of vitamin C is now recognized as a risk factor for suffering a heart attack or stroke. In one study involving over 6,600 men and women, those with the highest vitamin C levels enjoyed a 27 per cent lower risk of coronary heart disease and a 26 per cent lower risk of stroke than those with low levels. According to another study of 1,605 middle-aged men, those with vitamin C deficiency were 3.5 times more likely to have a heart attack than men with vitamin C levels above the deficiency level. Low levels of vitamin C are also linked with an increased risk of developing angina.

As vitamin C protects genetic material from damaging oxidation reactions, people with the highest intakes also enjoy the lowest risk of developing a number of cancers – especially when supplements are taken together with vitamin E and selenium. This is supported by a recent study in Norfolk, UK, involving over 19,000 adults aged 45 to 79 years, which found that circulating levels of vitamin C were inversely related to death from all causes over the four-year study period.

BENEFITS OF VITAMIN E

Vitamin E is an antioxidant that protects fatty parts of the body from damaging oxidation reactions. This slows the progression of atherosclerosis and reduces the risk of blood-clot formation. Men with the lowest intakes of vitamin E have the highest risk of angina, even after adjusting for age, blood pressure, cholesterol levels, weight and smoking.

Vitamin E gained widespread acceptance among doctors following results of the Cambridge Heart Antioxidant Study (CHAOS) in 1996. Just over 2,000 people with coronary heart disease were divided into two groups. Half took vitamin E for 18 months, while half received an inactive placebo. Taking high-dose vitamin E (at least 400iu daily) was found to reduce the risk of a heart attack by as much as 77 per cent. In fact, the protective effect was so strong, it seemed the group treated with vitamin E were at no greater risk of another heart attack than people who did not have coronary heart disease. As a result, many physicians now recommend high-dose vitamin E supplements for older people, especially those at risk of heart attack.

Other large trials have shown that both men and women can reduce their risk of ever developing coronary heart disease by as much as 40 per cent through taking vitamin E supplements – risk is lowest in those taking 100iu (around 67mg) of vitamin E per day for at least 2 years.

CAROTENOIDS

Carotenoids are yellow-orange-red pigments, of which over 600 are present in fruit and vegetables. Only a few, such as alphacarotene, betacarotene, lycopene, lutein and zeaxanthin, are currently recognized as important for human health. Lycopene – the red pigment in tomatoes – appears to be the most beneficial carotenoid for protecting against both coronary heart disease and cancer.

In a large, international study covering 10 countries in Europe, a significant link was found between low lycopene levels and increased risk of developing a first heart attack. An analysis of 72 studies also found that 57 reported significant links between tomato intake or blood lycopene levels and reduced risk of cancer, especially of the lung, stomach, mouth, colon, rectum and prostate gland. After accounting for smoking, people with the lowest levels of lycopene appear to be three times more likely to develop lung cancer than those with the highest intakes. It was recently reported that another carotenoid, lutein – mainly taken for its beneficial effects on the eyes – may also protect against the development of early atherosclerosis.

DOSE

Although diet should always come first, many experts now agree that food alone cannot supply the optimum quantities of antioxidants needed. A good multivitamin and mineral supplement supplying additional antioxidants is therefore a good idea.

Researchers have analysed blood levels of antioxidants in large numbers of people and followed them up to see who developed coronary heart disease and cancer. Those with the least risk of these diseases are those with the highest circulating levels of protective antioxidants. Guidelines for nutrient intake were defined as a means of preventing deficiencies such as scurvy. Modern evidence suggests we might benefit from higher intakes of antioxidant nutrients.

Those with high blood levels of the antioxidant vitamins C and E (usually through taking supplements) are three times less likely to have a heart attack than those with low levels. The following intakes are suggested:

* vitamin C: 120–1,000mg per day
* vitamin E: 25–250mg per day
* selenium 100–200mcg per day.

Lower doses may be appropriate for people taking other antioxidant sources such as alpha-lipoic acid, green tea, pycnogenol or grapeseed extracts.

People who smoke or who have diabetes generally need higher amounts of antioxidants than other people.

Calcium

Low intakes of calcium have been linked with an increased risk of high blood pressure and stroke. Your body contains more calcium than any other mineral. Ninety-nine per cent (around 1.2kg) is stored in your skeleton (bones and teeth), while the other 1 per cent (around 10g) plays a central role in functions like muscle contraction, nerve conduction, blood clotting, regulation of metabolic enzymes, energy production and immunity.

Foods containing calcium include:

* milk (semi-skimmed and skimmed milks actually contain slightly more calcium than full-fat and are better for your overall health)
* dairy products such as low-fat cheese, yoghurt, fromage frais
* green leafy vegetables such as broccoli
* salmon
* nuts and seeds
* pulses
* white and brown bread – in the UK, white and brown flour are fortified with calcium by law, but not wholemeal flour
* eggs.

The EC recommended daily intake for calcium is 800mg, although to prevent osteoporosis, some people need a daily intake of 1,000–1,500mg.

Lack of calcium is thought to affect the way your circulation responds to changes in blood pressure detected by receptors in blood vessel walls (baroreceptors) – perhaps by interfering with nerve signals to arterioles that encourage them to dilate. In fact, drugs that affect calcium channels in the body are highly successful in treating hypertension, angina, some irregular heart rhythms and poor circulation.

Calcium is absorbed in the small intestine, a process for which vitamin D is essential. Usually, less than 40 per cent of dietary calcium is absorbed from the gut – the remainder is lost in bowel motions. Some types of fibre (phytates from wheat in unleavened breads such as chapattis) bind calcium in the bowel to form an insoluble, non-absorbable salt. High-fibre diets, which speed the passage of food through the bowels, also reduce the amount of calcium absorbed. As a high-fibre diet is important for health, you need to ensure you have a good intake of calcium – even if this means taking supplements.

DOSE

Some experts recommend that someone with high blood pressure should consider taking a 1,000mg calcium supplement (plus magnesium, see below) with their evening meal (when calcium flux in your body is greatest) for two months to see if this produces a fall in BP.

Magnesium

Magnesium and calcium work together in the body. Low intakes of magnesium have also been linked with an increased risk of high blood pressure and stroke.

Seventy per cent of your body magnesium is stored in your bones and teeth, but its most important role is to maintain the integrity of your cells. Special salt pumps maintain different ion concentration gradients across cell walls – these are needed for the cell to act like a battery, holding an electric charge and passing electrical messages from one cell to another. Magnesium is essential for these membrane pumps and for maintaining each cell's electrical stability. It is especially important in controlling calcium entry into heart cells to trigger a regular heartbeat.

Magnesium is vital for every major metabolic reaction, from the synthesis of protein and genetic material to the production of energy from glucose. Few enzymes can work without it and magnesium is now known to be vital for healthy tissues, especially those of the muscles, lung airways, blood vessels and nerves. Researchers have found that people with low levels of magnesium are more at risk of spasm of the coronary arteries (linked with angina or heart attack) and spasm of airways, leading to asthma as well as high blood pressure.

Foods containing magnesium include:

* soya beans
* nuts
* brewer's yeast
* wholegrains
* wholewheat flour
* brown rice
* seafood
* meat
* eggs
* dairy products
* bananas
* dark green, leafy vegetables.

Food processing, however, removes most magnesium content. If you have high BP, a supplement containing magnesium is a good idea.

Dose

Take 150–500mg daily, preferably with food to optimize absorption. Magnesium citrate is most readily absorbed, while magnesium gluconate is less likely to cause intestinal side-effects such as diarrhoea at higher doses.

If taking magnesium supplements, ensure you also have a good intake of calcium.

Co-enzyme Q10

Co-enzyme Q10 (CoQ10) is a vitamin-like substance that improves oxygen utilization and energy production. It is needed to process oxygen in cells, and to generate energy-rich molecules. CoQ10 acts together with vitamin E to form a powerful antioxidant defence against oxidation damage to body fats, including those in the circulation. Like other antioxidants, CoQ10 seems to protect against hardening and furring up of the arteries (atherosclerosis) and to reduce the risk of heart disease.

After the age of about 20, levels of CoQ10 start to decrease as dietary CoQ10 is absorbed less efficiently from the intestines and its production in body cells starts to fall. Lack of CoQ10 mean that cells – including heart muscle cells – do not receive all the energy they need. They therefore function at a sub-optimal level and are more likely to become diseased and to age prematurely. Research suggests falling CoQ10 levels play a significant role in age-related medical conditions such as coronary heart disease.

Biopsies of heart muscles from patients with various forms of heart disease have shown that 50–75 per cent are deficient in CoQ10. It seems that CoQ10 reduces the size and stickiness of platelets – blood fragments involved in clotting – and may help to reduce the risk of abnormal blood clots that play a role in heart attack. At least one study has found that the more severe the heart disease, the lower the levels of CoQ10. Some doctors have therefore used CoQ10 to help treat patients with coronary heart disease and heart failure.

Supplements of CoQ10 have been used to normalize high blood pressure. In a trial involving 18 patients with essential hypertension, a daily dose of 100mg of CoQ10 was found to significantly reduce blood pressure compared with a placebo. Average systolic pressure fell by 10.6mmHg, and diastolic pressure by 7.7mmHg when taking CoQ10, but did not change with the placebo. CoQ10 is thought to lower hypertension by improving the elasticity and reactivity of the blood vessel wall.

In another trial involving 109 people with essential hypertension, an average daily dose of 225mg of CoQ10 was added to their existing drug regime. A significant, gradual improvement in BP occurred. Overall, 51 per cent of participants were able to stop between one and three anti-hypertensive drugs within 4.4 months of starting CoQ10. Those receiving echocardiograms showed a significant improvement in left ventricular wall thickness and function so heart pumping became more efficient. Only 3 per cent of patients required the addition of one anti-hypertensive drug.

DOSE

The optimal dietary intake of CoQ10 is unknown. Commercially available dietary supplements recommend 10–100mg CoQ10 daily, often taken as two separate doses. Higher doses of 300–600mg daily may be suggested to treat illnesses such as severe heart disease and high blood pressure under medical supervision.

CoQ10 is fat-soluble and best taken with food to improve absorption. It usually takes at least three weeks, and occasionally up to three months, before the full beneficial effect and extra energy levels are noticed.

No serious side-effects or long-term problems have been reported, even at high doses – only occasional and transient mild nausea.

Hawthorn (*Crategus oxycantha* and *C. monogyna*)

The flowering tops and berries of the hawthorn are one of the most beneficial herbal remedies available for hypertension. Hawthorn helps to reduce high blood pressure by relaxing peripheral blood vessels and dilating coronary arteries through its ability to block the action of an enzyme (ACE or angiotensin-converting enzyme), which improves blood circulation to the heart muscle and the peripheries. It also has a mild diuretic action, which discourages fluid retention, and can also slow or possibly even reverse the build-up of atheromatous plaques to reduce hardening and furring up of the arteries (atherosclerosis). Hawthorn extracts also increase the strength and efficiency of the heart's pumping action. These actions have been shown to reduce shortness of breath, ankle oedema (swelling) and increase exercise tolerance in people with heart problems compared with those taking a placebo.

Other beneficial actions include promoting calm, reducing stress and overcoming insomnia.

Dose

100–450mg daily (standardized to at least 1.8 per cent vitexin). Larger amounts are usually divided between three doses.

Hawthorn extracts may take up to two months to show an appreciable effect. Side-effects are rare, although nausea, sweating and skin rashes have been reported. If you suffer from a heart condition, check with your doctor before taking it, especially if you are on prescribed medication.

Dandelion (*Taraxacum officinalis*)

This well-known weed is used for its detoxifying properties. Dandelion leaf is used for its diuretic action on the kidneys, helping to increase the elimination of water-soluble toxins from the body. Dandelion also has a useful mineral content, including potassium, which helps to flush excess sodium through the kidneys. This makes it an excellent treatment for water retention and hypertension as it can reduce fluid retention without also encouraging a build-up of sodium. Interestingly, dandelion does not seem to have a diuretic action in those with a normal, healthy fluid balance who do not need to lose excess water.

Dose

5–10g of fresh root daily, divided between two or three doses. Or 500mg of dandelion extract twice a day.

Side-effects are uncommon, but large doses can cause nausea and diarrhoea. Do not use if you have active gallstones or obstructive jaundice.

Ginkgo (*Ginkgo biloba*)

Ginkgo is one of the most popular health supplements in Europe. Its fan-shaped leaves contain a variety of powerful antioxidants, flavoglycosides, bioflavones and unique chemicals known as ginkgolides and bilobalides. These have been found to relax blood vessels in the body and boost blood circulation to the brain, hands, feet and genitals by stopping cell fragments in the blood (platelets) from clumping together. Many people find it helps to improve memory and concentration, as well as easing dizziness and improving their peripheral circulation – problems which can accompany long-standing high blood pressure and atherosclerosis.

Dose

Extracts standardized for at least 24 per cent ginkgolides: 40–60mg two to three times a day. One-a-day formulations are also available. Take a minimum of 120mg daily. Effects may not be noticed until after 10 days' treatment and may take up to 12 weeks to produce a noticeable benefit.

A handful of cases have appeared in the medical literature in which bleeding within the skull (subarachnoid haemorrhage or subdural haematoma) have occurred in people taking Ginkgo biloba extracts in combination with warfarin (a powerful blood-thinning drug) or aspirin. Although ginkgolides found in Ginkgo biloba do inhibit platelet aggregation, these are present in small concentrations and, at usual therapeutic doses of Ginkgo biloba, no effects on platelet aggregation have been found. Certainly, in people not taking blood-thinning agents, there appears to be no cause for concern.

In a double-blind, placebo-controlled, randomized trial of Ginkgo biloba extracts in dementia, the one subdural haematoma that occurred out of 309 patients was in the placebo group. For people taking warfarin or aspirin, however, it is best to err on the side of caution and to avoid using Ginkgo biloba until any possible interactions have been fully investigated.

Do not use unprocessed Ginkgo leaves (such as from garden trees) as these contain powerful chemicals that can cause allergic reactions.

Padma 28

An interesting Tibetan preparation, Padma 28 contains a complex mix of 20 Tibetan medicinal herbs that are helpful against intermittent claudication (*see Chapter 2*). Padma 28 is currently undergoing trials at the London Middlesex Hospital as it has previously been shown in a pilot clinical trial to increase pain-free walking distance in over half of patients.

Choline and Phosphatidyl-choline (Lecithin)

Choline is an essential, vitamin-like substance, most of which is obtained from the diet in the form of phosphatidyl-choline (lecithin). Choline and lecithin act as emulsifiers to help break down dietary fats into smaller particles that can be absorbed and used in the body.

Supplements appear to reduce the risk of coronary heart disease (CHD) by lowering abnormal cholesterol levels. They do this by inhibiting intestinal absorption of cholesterol and increasing excretion of cholesterol in bile. In one study involving 32 people with high blood lipids who took 10.5g of lecithin for 30 days, average total cholesterol and triglycerides decreased by one-third, harmful LDL-cholesterol decreased by 38 per cent and beneficial HDL-cholesterol increased by 46 per cent. The researchers concluded that lecithin should be administered for the prevention and treatment of atherosclerosis.

Choline may also reduce the risk of CHD by boosting metabolism of homocysteine, an amino acid strongly linked with increased risk of circulatory problems (*see Chapter 6*).

Dose

Choline: 100–500mg daily.
Phosphatidylcholine (capsules): 1–2g daily, usually divided into three doses.

High doses of choline (e.g. 10g daily) can cause indigestion, anorexia, sweating and, over time, nerve and cardiovascular distress as well as a strong, fishy body odour. Lecithin supplements are therefore generally preferred. They are best taken with meals to boost absorption.

Supplements should not be taken by those with manic depression, except under medical supervision, in case it makes their condition worse.

L-Carnitine

L-carnitine is a non-essential amino acid made in the liver. It recently hit the headlines when it was reported that, taken together with alpha-lipoic acid – a vitamin-like antioxidant that acts as a co-enzyme to speed energy production in the body – it had anti-ageing properties.

Its most important role is in regulating fat metabolism. It is needed to transport long-chain fatty acids into the energy-producing mitochondria found in all body cells where they are burned to produce energy. The more L-carnitine available, the more fat can be utilized. This is especially so in heart muscle cells, which can be damaged if they do not receive enough oxygen or energy as metabolism is impaired and free fatty acids accumulate. Research suggests that L-carnitine helps to neutralize these fatty acids but may quickly become used up, so taking supplements is beneficial.

Providing additional L-carnitine may help minimize heart damage in those at risk of a heart attack. L-carnitine is also needed to break down the branched-chain amino acids (leucine, isoleucine and valine) so they can be used as an energy source by muscle cells when other sources of energy are in short supply. Among a group of 44 men with angina, almost 23 per cent who took L-carnitine supplements for four weeks became free of exercise-induced angina, compared with only 9 per cent taking an inactive placebo.

L-carnitine has been shown to improve the distance walked without pain by patients with calf pain (intermittent claudication) due to hardening and furring up of the arteries (atherosclerosis). In one study, 2g of L-carnitine taken twice daily allowed pain-free walking distance to increase by 75 per cent after three weeks of supplementation due to improved energy metabolism within muscle cells.

Dose

250mg to 1g daily.

Diarrhoea may occur at very high doses (more than 4g daily).

Increased body odour can occur when taking higher doses.

L-carnitine and co-enzyme Q10 seem to work synergistically.

If you have a medical disorder or are on prescription drugs, seek advice from a nutritional therapist before taking L-carnitine.

Flaxseed Oil (*Linum usitatissimum*)

Flaxseed oil is the richest-known plant source of an omega-3 essential fatty acid (alpha-linolenic acid) similar to the essential fatty acids (EFAs) found in fish oil, but less potent. For those who are allergic to fish, or who don't like fishy burps, flaxseed oil is a good alternative. Flaxseed oil also contains a beneficial omega-6 essential fatty acid, linoleic acid.

Flaxseed oil has beneficial effects on circulating blood fats, including LDL-cholesterol, and is widely recommended for people with coronary heart disease and high blood pressure. Some evidence suggests that, as with fish oils, if taken by those who have had a heart attack, it may reduce the chance of a second heart attack occurring.

Dose

1 teaspoon to 1 tablespoon, once or twice a day.

Flaxseeds: 1–2 tablespoons with water, twice a day.

Best taken with food to enhance absorption.

Hemp Seed Oil (*Cannabis sativa*)

Oil from the seed of the non-drug strain of cannabis, known as the hemp plant, contains both omega-6 and omega-3 essential fatty acids in a ratio of three to one, which includes gammalinolenic acid (GLA). Hemp seed oil has similar uses to evening primrose, flaxseed and omega-3 fish oils, and can help maintain a healthy circulation.

Dose

5–15ml daily, best taken with food.

Hemp seed oil supplements do not contain the psycho-active chemical (tetrahydrocannabinol) found in other (marijuana) strains of the cannabis plant.

Bilberry (*Vaccinium myrtillus*)

Bilberries are a rich source of tannins, anthocyanins and flavonoid glycosides that have powerful antioxidant and anti-inflammatory properties. Extracts are widely used to strengthen blood vessels and the collagen-containing connective tissue that supports them, as well as improving circulation. It appears to reduce the risk of stroke and inhibit unwanted clot formation. The beneficial effects on small blood vessels are especially apparent in the eye, and are used to help treat a number of eye problems, including the retinal changes associated with advanced hypertension.

Bilberry's effectiveness in treating visual problems results from a number of actions. Its antioxidant blue-red pigments:

* protect the membranes of light-sensitive and other cells in the eyes
* reduce hardening and furring up of blood vessels
* stabilize tear production
* increase blood flow to the retina
* regenerate the light-sensitive pigment, rhodopsin
* increase the strength of collagen fibres in capillaries and supportive connective tissues.

Visual acuity can improve in some cases by over 80 per cent within just 15 days.

Bilberry also contains a unique anthocyanoside, myrtillin, which helps to lower a raised blood sugar level through a similar action to insulin.

Dose

20–60g dried ripe fruit daily.

Dry extract (25 per cent anthocyanosides): 80–160mg, three times daily. Those with diabetes may be advised to take more than this.

No toxicity has been found, even at high doses, as bilberry is water-soluble and excess is quickly excreted through the urine and bile.

Royal Jelly

Royal jelly is a milky-white substance – also known as bee's milk – secreted in the salivary glands of worker honey bees. It is one of the richest natural sources of vitamin B5 (pantothenic acid), and also contains other B-vitamins plus vitamins A, C, D and E, 20 amino acids, essential fatty acids, minerals such as potassium, calcium, zinc, iron and manganese plus acetylcholine – a neuro-transmitter needed to transmit messages from one nerve cell to another.

Royal jelly is traditionally taken to boost energy levels and as a tonic to increase vitality. It may help to protect against hardening and furring up of the arteries by lowering total blood fats and abnormal cholesterol levels. Doses of 50–100mg of royal jelly per day were found to decrease total cholesterol levels by 14 per cent and total blood lipids by 10 per cent – possibly by increasing cholesterol excretion in the bile and decreasing its reabsorption in the gastrointestinal tract so less enters the circulation.

Dose

Typically 50–100mg per day.

Freeze-dried royal jelly blended with honey is available. Royal jelly supplements should be kept refrigerated and taken on an empty stomach.

Royal jelly has been known to trigger severe asthma attacks in some people with asthma so do not take if you are allergic to bee products, or if you suffer from asthma or other allergic conditions.

Specialist Herbal Medicines

A number of more specialist herbal medicines may be prescribed by a qualified herbal practitioner. These are not all widely available over the counter, although some – such as valerian – are becoming more popular in general use. If you wish to try one of the more powerful remedies described below, it is usually advisable to have them individually prescribed by a herbal practitioner, or a pharmacist.

ASTRAGALUS MEMBRANACEUS

Astragalus root (Huang Qi) is used in Chinese medicine as a cardiotonic and diuretic, sometimes recommended in the treatment of high blood pressure.

BLACK HAW (VIBURNUM PRUNIFOLIUM)

Dried bark from black haw, a close relative of cramp bark, helps to relax muscle tension and also has sedative actions, both of which explain its ability to lower blood pressure.

BUCKWHEAT (FAGOPYRUM ESCULENTUM)

Buckwheat leaves are traditionally used to improve the tone of arteriolar walls and to help repair damage that may lead to atherosclerosis. It is sometimes used in the treatment of high blood pressure, especially that linked with retinal haemorrhage.

BUGLEWEED (*LYCOPUS EUROPAEUS*)

The leaves, stems and flowers of bugleweed increase the power of heart muscle contractions, reduce the pulse rate and have a diuretic action. It is mainly used to treat heart failure, especially where this is due to high blood pressure or an over-active thyroid gland. It is also used as a sedative and anti-cough remedy.

CHRYSANTHEMUM (*CHRYSANTHEMUM MORIFOLIUM*)

Chrysanthemum flowers (Ju Hua) are used in Chinese medicine to dilate the coronary arteries, improve blood flow through the heart muscle and boost cardiac output. As heart function improves, treatment can reduce and stabilize high blood pressure.

CRAMP BARK (*VIBURNUM OPULUS*)

As its name suggests, cramp bark (the guelder rose) is used to reduce muscle tension and spasm. This relaxant action also occurs in smooth muscles lining peripheral blood vessels. It also has a sedative action that can lessen the effects of stress. Both actions help to reduce high blood pressure.

HORSETAIL (*EQUISETUM ARVENSE*)

The dried stems of horsetail have a mild diuretic action and may be used to reduce fluid retention.

LEMON BALM (*MELISSA OFFICINALIS*)

Lemon balm is a healing herb with calming properties. Its leaves are widely used to combat the effects of nervous stress, to improve heart function and to lower blood pressure.

LILY OF THE VALLEY (*CONVALLARIA MAJALIS*)

Dried lily of the valley leaves contain a number of powerful cardiac glycosides, two of which act directly on the heart. They have a similar action to digitoxin (from the foxglove) but without the potentially dangerous side-effects. Lily of the valley is used to help treat angina, hardening and furring up of the arteries (atherosclerosis), water retention due to heart failure and heart failure associated with high blood pressure.

LIME BLOSSOM (*TILIA VULGARIS*)

Dried flowers from the lime blossom, or linden tree, have an anti-atheroma action similar to that of garlic. With long-term use it can help to prevent furring up of the arteries and may even reduce the amount of atheroma already present. It is widely used to lower high blood pressure and to reduce the effects of nervous tension. Its anti-hypertensive effect seems to be due to relaxation and dilation of blood vessels.

MISTLETOE (*VISCUM ALBA*)

Mistletoe leaves and twigs (not the berries, which are poisonous) have a direct action on the vagus nerve (a cranial nerve stretching from the brain down to the heart and chest) to slow the heart rate. It also strengthens the walls of small blood vessels (capillaries) and helps combat atherosclerosis. It can lower blood pressure significantly, and is also used to ease headaches associated with high BP.

MOTHERWORT (*LEONURUS CARDIACA*)
The leaves of motherwort have been used since Roman times to strengthen the heart muscle, ease palpitations, regulate a fast pulse and to lower a raised blood pressure. Motherwort is also used to ease anxiety and nervous tension.

NIGHT-BLOOMING CEREUS (*SELENICEREUS GRANDIFLORUS*)
Fresh stems from the night-blooming cereus have a similar action on the heart to lily of the valley. It is used to treat mild heart failure, water retention, shortness of breath and palpitations. It does not contain cardiac glycosides.

PAEONY (*PAEONIA SPP.*)
Paeony root is used to stimulate the circulation, reduce high blood pressure, relieve pain and for its sedative action.

SKULLCAP (*SCUTELLARIA LATERIFOLIA*)
Leaves and flowers from the skullcap are widely used to treat stress and related problems including nervous tension, hysteria, exhaustion and depression. It can help to lower high blood pressure linked with acute stress.

SQUILL (*URGINEA MARITIMA*)
Squill contains cardiac glycosides that stimulate the heart and is used to help treat congestive heart failure and associated water retention (e.g. secondary to high blood pressure). Only a minute quantity of the bulb is prescribed and this is usually given in the form of a dilute tincture.

VALERIAN (*VALERIANA OFFICINALIS*)
The natural sedative found in valerian roots makes this one of the most relaxing herbs available. It has significant, positive effects on stress and, as well as relieving anxiety and tension, induces sleep, eases smooth muscle spasm and promotes calmness. It is used to lower high blood pressure, especially when linked with stress.

WOOD BETONY (*STACHYS OFFICINALIS*)
The leaves, stems and flowers of wood betony have a sedative action and are used to treat nervous tension. It is a relaxant and painkiller useful for treating tension headache linked with stress and raised blood pressure.

YARROW (*ACHILLEA MILLEFOLIUM*)
The leaves, stems and flowers of yarrow contain chemicals that lower raised blood pressure by encouraging the dilation of peripheral blood vessels, and through a diuretic action. It also has an anti-atheroma action and is commonly recommended to help treat thrombotic conditions linked with high blood pressure.

CHAPTER 20

High Blood Pressure and Healthy Weight

Being overweight significantly increases your risk of many diseases, including high blood pressure, coronary heart disease and stroke. Having to pump blood through excess fatty tissues increases the workload of the heart, and people who are overweight are also more likely to eat excess fat, have high blood cholesterol and glucose levels, and have low levels of physical activity. All these factors hasten atherosclerosis and are associated with hypertension.

Doctors may soon be able to predict which people with hypertension will respond best to losing weight by measuring their blood levels of circulating renin. This hormone is made in the kidneys and acts to put blood pressure up. For people with high renin levels, weight loss seems to be three times more effective in reducing blood pressure than in those with low renin levels. They also respond better to a low-sodium, high-potassium diet.

Are You a Healthy Weight for Your Height?
The most accurate way of working out if you are in the healthy weight range for your height is to calculate your body mass index (BMI). You do this by dividing your weight (in kilograms) by the square of your height (in metres).

$$BMI = \frac{\text{Weight (kg)}}{\text{Height x Height (m}^2\text{)}}$$

The calculation produces a number that can be interpreted by the following table:

BMI	Weight Band
<20	Underweight
20–25	Healthy
25–30	Overweight
30–40	Obese
>40	Morbidly obese

A BMI of 20–25 is in the healthy weight range as it is not linked with an increased risk of early death. A slightly stricter range applies for women. The following chart shows the healthy weight ranges for your particular height (based on BMI 18.7–23.8 for women, and BMI 20–25 for men).

HEIGHT   OPTIMUM HEALTHY WEIGHT RANGE

| MEN | | | WOMEN | |
Metres (Feet)	Kilos	Stones	Kilos	Stones
1.47 (4'10")			40–51	6st 4–8st
1.50 (4'11")			42–54	6st 8–8st 7
1.52 (5')			43–55	6st 11–8st 9
1.55 (5'1")			45–57	7st 1–8st 13
1.57 (5'2")			46–59	7st 3–9st 4
1.60 (5'3")			48–61	7st 8–9st 8
1.63 (5'4")			50–63	7st 12–9st 13
1.65 (5'5")			51–65	8st–10st 3
1.68 (5'6")	56–70	8st 12–11 st	53–67	8st 5–10st 7
1.70 (5'7")	58–72	9st 1–11st 4	54–69	8st 7–10st 12
1.73 (5'8")	60–75	9st 6–11st 10	56–71	8st 11–11st 2
1.75 (5'9")	61–76	9st 9–12 st	57–73	8st 13–11st 7
1.78 (5'10")	63–79	9st 13–12st 6	59–75	9st 4–11st 11
1.80 (5'11")	65–81	10st 3–12st 9	61–77	9st 8–12st 1
1.83 (6')	67–83	10st 7–13st 1	63–80	9st 13–12st 8
1.85 (6'1")	69–85	10st 11–13st 5		
1.88 (6'2")	71–88	11st 2–13st 12		
1.90 (6'3")	72–90	11st 5–14st 2		
1.93 (6'4")	75–93	11st 10–14st 8		

If your BMI falls above this range, you are either overweight (BMI of 25–30) or obese (BMI of 30–40 or more). Being overweight increases your risk of premature death from high blood pressure, CHD or stroke by 50 per cent. If you are obese, your risk of premature death from these causes is double that of someone who is in the healthy weight range for their height.

If you are overweight, where you store your excess fat is also important. Those who carry excess weight around their middle (apple-shaped) rather than around their hips (pear-shaped) are more at risk of a number of conditions, including diabetes, atherosclerosis, coronary heart disease, high blood pressure and stroke. The exact reason is unknown, but is probably due to the genes that dictate how your body handles dietary fats.

To work out if you are apple-shaped, measure your waist and hips in centimetres using a non-stretchable tape measure. Divide your waist measurement by your hip measurement to get your waist/hip ratio. A waist/hip ratio greater than 0.85 is apple-shaped for women, while a ratio greater than 0.95 is apple-shaped for males.

Waist size alone may also be a good indicator as research suggests men with a waist circumference larger than 102cm and women with a waist circumference larger than 88cm are more likely to develop diabetes and hypertension than those who are slimmer. Slight waist reductions of just 5–10cm have been shown to significantly reduce the risk of a heart attack, so try to lose any excess weight by following a sensible low-fat diet and increasing your level of physical activity. The good news is that fat stored on the abdomen seems to be easier to shift than fat stored on the hips.

If you are overweight and apple shaped as well, you have a significantly high risk of developing high blood pressure and coronary heart disease and should seriously consider losing at least some of your excess fat. Just shedding half a stone can produce a significant fall in high blood pressure.

How to Lose Weight

The only way to lose weight is to eat fewer calories than you burn. The most successful way to do this is to lose only around 0.5–1kg (1–2lb) per week. If you try to lose weight more quickly, your health may suffer. You are also less likely to lose weight and keep it off – your metabolism is designed to conserve energy in the face of possible impending starvation and will slow right down, so you shed excess fat more slowly and painfully. Once you start eating normally again, your metabolism will stay on its super-efficient setting and the weight will pile back on.

Most experts now agree that you need to:

* follow a low-fat diet to remove excess weight
* exercise regularly to keep the weight off.

To lose weight, follow a healthy, low-fat diet, increase your intake of fruit and vegetables, and step up the amount of physical exercise you take (*see Chapter 21*). You may find it helpful to join a slimming club to provide motivation and useful low-fat, healthy-eating advice.

You can reduce the amount of fat you eat by adopting the following recommended food preparation and cooking methods. These techniques have the added bonus of increasing the nutrient value of your food:

* Eat fruit and vegetables raw or only lightly steamed.
* Grill (broil) food with only a light brushing of olive or rapeseed oil.
* Bake.
* Boil with only minimal amounts of water and no added salt or bicarbonate of soda.
* Poaching in vegetable stock (Court Bouillon)
* Stir-fry using a light brushing of olive or rapeseed oil.
* If roasting meat, place the meat on a rack within the roasting pan so all the juices and fats drain away. When roasting chicken, use a glass funnel roaster onto which you prop the chicken vertically in the oven. All the fats will then drain off so you are left with beautifully flavoured, low-fat meat.
* When making gravy to go with the roast, ensure it's low in fat and rich in nutrients by using gravy granules plus the water your vegetables were cooked in.
* To make a low-fat dressing or sauce for salads, fish and meat, use low-fat yoghurt or fromage frais with herbs, tomato juice, orange/lemon juice and black pepper.

Tips to Help You Eat Less

* Drink a large glass of sparkling mineral water before every meal – this will make you feel full more quickly so you eat less.
* If possible, try to eat the main meal of the day at lunchtime – your metabolic rate is higher than in the evening, so more calories are burned than converted into fat. Try not to eat after 6pm at night.
* Always sit down at a laid table – don't eat while standing up.
* Serve smaller helpings than you think you need.
* Use a smaller plate than usual.
* Eat more complex, unrefined carbohydrates (e.g. brown rice, wholegrain cereals, wholegrain bread, wholewheat pasta etc) – these contain complex carbohydrates that trigger the release of serotonin in the brain, making you feel fuller more quickly.
* Eat as slowly as possible, so that metabolic messages that you are full start to come through before you have finished your food.
  · Chew each mouthful longer than usual.
  · Pause regularly while eating and put down your knife and fork between bites.
  · Rediscover the art of mealtime conversation.
* Concentrate on enjoying your food. Don't read or watch television at the same time – you will swallow mechanically without appreciating your food and end up eating more.
* Try not to eat while driving – this can become a habit on long journeys.
* Use low-calorie versions of everything possible when cooking or eating. Skimmed milk has almost 50 per cent fewer calories per pint than whole milk. On an allowance of half a pint per day, you can save 450 calories a week.
* Cut down on cooking fats. Don't roast or deep-fry. Instead, grill (broil), bake or stir-fry using a non-stick pan.
* Low-fat yoghurt is an ideal substitute for cream in most recipes (NB It will curdle if you let it
* boil.)
* When you feel the urge to eat between meals, do some vigorous exercise and work up a sweat – or try cleaning your teeth with strong, tingling toothpaste.
* If the scales refuse to budge, keep a food diary and write down everything you eat.

Chapter 21

High Blood Pressure and Lifestyle

Lifestyle habits such as alcohol intake (*see Chapter 11*), smoking, stress levels, physical activity and using relaxation techniques all influence your long-term blood pressure. As we will see in this chapter, making lifestyle changes can help reduce hypertension.

Smoking

Smoking cigarettes is linked with early death from a number of illnesses, including coronary heart disease, high blood pressure and stroke. If you can give up, however, your health will quickly benefit:

* Within 20 minutes: your blood pressure and pulse rate will fall significantly as arterial spasm decreases.
* Within eight hours: levels of carbon monoxide in your blood drop to normal so that blood oxygen levels can rise.
* Within 48 hours: the stickiness of your blood and the quantity of blood-clotting factors present will fall enough to reduce your risk of a heart attack or stroke.
* Within one to three months: the blood supply to your peripheral circulation will increase, and your lung function will improve by up to a third
* Within five years: your risk of lung cancer will have halved.
* Within 10 years: your risk of all smoking-related cancers (such as lung, mouth, throat, bladder) will have reduced to almost normal levels.

TIPS ON HOW TO STOP SMOKING
* Get into the right frame of mind.
* Name the day to give up.
* Try to stop at the same time as a friend or relative for support.
* Throw away all smoking bits and pieces such as matches, lighters and ashtrays.
* Take it one day at a time and just concentrate on getting through each day.
* Keep a chart and tick off each successful day.
* Find something to occupy your hands – make models, try drawing or origami.
* Take extra exercise.

- When you have an urge to smoke, try sucking on celery or carrot sticks, eating an apple, or cleaning your teeth with strong-flavoured toothpaste.
- Avoid situations where you used to smoke.
- Learn to say 'No thanks, I've given up.'
- Ask friends and relatives not to smoke around you.

Stress

Stress is the term used to describe being under too much pressure. A certain amount of stress is good for you and helps you meet life's challenges. It is only when stress exceeds your perceived ability to cope that it becomes harmful, as when you feel under excess pressure, your pulse and blood pressure rise significantly. One study involving almost 300 male employees in America, found those reporting high levels of work stress had blood pressure raised by an equivalent amount to carrying an extra 40lb in weight, or an additional 20 years in age. In some people, stress can trigger overactivity of the sympathetic nervous system, causing large daily swings in blood-pressure measurements. This is known as *labile hypertension* or *Gaisbock's syndrome* (*see Chapter 2*), and can increase your risk of developing future sustained hypertension and of suffering a stroke.

Stress is also harmful because it can trigger arterial spasm, chest pain, an irregular heart rhythm, angina and a heart attack. If you suffer from hypertension, it is important to reduce your stress levels.

TIPS TO HELP OVERCOME STRESS
- Keep a stress diary to help you work out what is making you stressed and why – change those situations that can be changed and, where practical, avoid others (such as shopping in the supermarket at the busiest times).
- Leave more time for tasks so they aren't done under deadline pressure.
- Learn to say 'no' so you aren't put upon by others.
- Try floatation therapy (*see page 177*).
- Increase your intake of vitamin C and the B-group as these are rapidly used up by stress reactions in your body.
- Cut back on sugar, salt and excess fat.
- Eat little and often to keep your blood sugar constant.
- If you smoke, try to cut back or stop.
- Keep alcohol intake within the low-risk range (*see page 61*).
- Avoid drinks and products containing high amounts of caffeine.
- Exercise regularly to burn off stress hormones.

The Health Benefits of Exercise

One of the most successful lifestyle changes you can make to lower high blood pressure is to increase the amount of exercise you take. This can lower your diastolic BP by around 10mmHg – similar to the effect of many anti-hypertensive drugs. Taking regular exercise can also lower several other factors linked with increased risk of high blood pressure and coronary heart disease. A study of more than 10,000 men found that exercise reduced the number of age-related deaths from all causes by almost a quarter, even if exercise was not started until middle age. Deaths from coronary heart disease (CHD) were reduced by 41 per cent, independent of other risk factors such as being overweight, high blood pressure or smoking cigarettes.

Exercise has also been shown to reduce your risk of a stroke by up to 50 per cent, and to reduce your risk of diabetes by up to 40 per cent. Research suggests that regular brisk exercise can reduce the risk of premature death from all causes by 23 per cent. It is best to join a gym to obtain individually tailored advice.

Ideally, you need to exercise briskly – enough to raise your pulse level to 110–120 per minute, work up a light sweat and leave you slightly breathless – for at least 30 minutes, at least five days a week, and preferably seven. Unfortunately, an estimated seven out of ten men, and eight out of ten women do not take enough exercise to reduce their risk of a heart attack. NB If you are seeing your doctor because of high blood pressure or heart problems, be guided by them as to the amount and level of exercise you should take.

WHY EXERCISE PROTECTS AGAINST CORONARY HEART DISEASE

Exercise protects the heart in a number of ways. It lowers harmful blood cholesterol levels and blood pressure, reduces hardening and furring up of the arteries and also improves the circulation of blood to the heart through small, collateral arteries.

The effect on blood fats is quite marked. In one study, volunteers were fed a high-fat meal of cereal, fruit and cream, which provided 66 per cent of calories in the form of fat. Blood samples were taken at regular intervals over the next six hours and blood fat levels analysed. When the subjects indulged in a prolonged bout of brisk walking, their blood fat levels rose much less than usual. This effect was noticed when exercise was taken as much as 15 hours before the meal, and when exercise was taken 90 minutes after the meal.

If you suffer from hypertension, you should consider starting a gentle, regular exercise programme today. You don't have to overdo it. Heart specialists in Australia followed 500 men who took either light exercise on a bicycle, steps and rowing machine with plenty of rests, or who continuously jogged or walked for 30 minutes. After a year, both groups were declared equally fit during treadmill tests.

HOW TO START AN EXERCISE REGIME

It is important to start your exercise programme slowly and carefully. If, after years of inactivity, you suddenly take up jogging or squash, you will be putting your heart under unnecessary strain. People starting an exercise programme too vigorously are likely to tear muscles or ligaments, damage joints and end up stiff, sore and lose motivation. You need to start slowly and increase your exercise levels gently and sensibly as your fitness level improves. To achieve fitness, start by taking regular exercise lasting at least 20 minutes, for a minimum of three times per week. Once you have achieved a reasonable level of fitness, you should do more.

* If you are unfit, start slowly and build up the time and effort you spend on exercise.
* Don't eat a heavy meal within two hours of exercise, either before or after.

- Make sure you wear loose clothing and proper footwear.
- Always warm up first with a few simple bends and stretches.
- Cool down afterwards by walking slowly for a few minutes.
- Stop if you feel dizzy, very short of breath, break into a cold sweat or get any pain.
- Avoid isolated places.
- If out at night, make sure you are fully visible near traffic.

If you have problems with your joints (such as arthritis) or find it difficult to manage a brisk walk, try a non-weight-bearing form of exercise such as cycling or swimming.

WALKING YOURSELF FIT

Brisk walking is an excellent exercise for building up your cardiovascular fitness. Swing your arms and put as much effort into your walking as possible. Begin slowly and lengthen your strides as you go. You should soon feel warm and start to generate a light sweat. Don't let yourself feel out of breath to the extent that you can't walk and talk at the same time. After your brisk walk, stroll gently for a few minutes to cool down, then do some simple stretching exercises to maintain muscle suppleness.

A suggested walking-for-fitness regime is given below. Obviously, you don't need to stick to the days of the week suggested, but try to spread your activity evenly throughout the week. If you find you can comfortably walk briskly for longer than the exercise periods suggested, then increase the time you spend and the distance covered to fast-track your way to fitness and better health.

Week	Tuesday	Thursday	Saturday	Sunday
1	10 mins	10 mins	15 mins	
2	10 mins	10 mins	15 mins	
3	10 mins	15 mins	15 mins	
4	15 mins	15 mins	15 mins	15 mins
5	15 mins	15 mins	20 mins	20 mins
6	20 mins	20 mins	25 mins	25 mins
7	25 mins	25 mins	25 mins	25 mins
8	30 mins	30 mins	30 mins	30 mins
9	30 mins	35 mins	30 mins	35 mins
10	40 mins	35 mins	40 mins	35 mins
11	40 mins	40 mins	40 mins	40 mins
12	45 mins	40 mins	45 mins	40 mins

If at any time you feel you have reached your comfortable exercise level and do not fancy walking any further, then stick at that level. After a while, when you feel like walking further, slowly build up your workout at your own pace.

To maintain your new fitness level, continue walking briskly three or four times per week. Try to obtain at least 30 minutes' exercise three times per week.

Relaxation Techniques

A number of relaxation techniques are helpful for reducing stress levels and helping to bring down a raised blood pressure.

TRANSCENDENTAL MEDITATION

Meditation uses a variety of mental techniques to attain a state of complete relaxation. The form known as transcendental meditation (TM) was developed by Maharishi Mahesh Yogi to be easily practised (15–20 minutes twice a day), despite our busy modern lifestyles. TM uses a variety of Sanskrit mantras, each of which is a short word or phrase that, when repeated in the mind, helps the user still their thoughts and find a deeper level of consciousness. This helps you achieve a deep relaxation, while alertness is fully maintained. It leaves you feeling mentally and physically refreshed, with a mind that is calmer and able to think more clearly. A study in *Hypertension – the Journal of the American Heart Association* showed that TM reduced systolic blood pressure by an average of 11mmHg and diastolic BP by 6mmHg within three months. It also reduces stress, anxiety and a raised cholesterol level, and improves quality of sleep, as well as helping people cut down on or stop smoking, alcohol consumption or drug abuse.

AROMATHERAPY

Essential oils used in aromatherapy have powerful effects on mood. The part of the brain that detects smell messages from the nose is closely linked with your emotional centre in a part of the brain called the limbic system. Oils are also absorbed from the skin into the circulation and can have powerful effects on the body. This is particularly noticeable with some that have diuretic properties.

Unless otherwise stated, aromatherapy oils should always be used in a diluted form by adding to a carrier oil, as some neat oils will irritate tissues. Use to massage into the skin, add to bath water or diffuse into the air to scent your room.

Avoid using aromatherapy oils that are known to be capable of putting blood pressure up. These include thyme, clove and cinnamon.

Essential oils that are used to help lower high blood pressure include:

* clary sage
* geranium
* lavender
* lemon
* marjoram
* melissa
* nutmeg
* rosemary
* ylang ylang.

Essential oils that have relaxing properties include:

* chamomile
* clary sage
* jasmine
* marjoram
* nutmeg
* pettigrain
* rose
* vetivert.

When making your own essential oil blends, add 1 drop of essential oil per 5ml (1 medicinal teaspoon) to make a 1 per cent solution. For larger quantities:
Add 10 drops of essential oil to 100ml carrier oil to produce a 0.5 per cent solution.
Add a total of 20 drops of essential oil to 100ml carrier oil to produce a 1 per cent solution.
Add a total of 40 drops of essential oil to 100ml carrier oil to produce a 2 per cent solution.
Suitable carrier oils include jojoba, almond, grapeseed, avocado, sunflower and wheatgerm.

FLOATATION THERAPY

This popular alternative therapy, which can trigger profound relaxation, takes place in a light-proof, sound-insulated tank. This contains a pool of warm water 10 inches deep in which 700lb of Epsom salts (magnesium sulphate) are dissolved to form a super-saturated solution more buoyant than the Dead Sea. The floater is suspended on this bed of minerals, which is kept at a constant skin temperature of 34.5°C. The tank is specially designed to screen out light and sound so the brain is cut off from virtually all external sources of stimulation – even the effects of gravity are minimized. This is probably important as it has been suggested that 90 per cent of all brain activity is concerned with the effects of gravitational pull on the body (such as correcting posture and maintaining balance).

Many physiological changes occur throughout the body during floatation, including a significant fall in blood pressure in both normal and hypertensive people. A number of mechanisms are probably at work in producing this fall:

* Blood levels of stress-inducing hormones (adrenaline, noradrenaline, cortisol and adrenocorticotrophic hormone) are reduced during repeated floatation sessions – this reduction is maintained even five days after treatment has stopped.
* The parasympathetic nervous system is activated, which reduces heart rate, blood pressure, respiratory rate and sweating, as well as relaxing muscles (including those in the arteries and arteriolar walls) and reducing oxygen requirements – these effects are opposite to those of the flight-and-fight (adrenaline) response linked with the sympathetic nervous system.
* Secretion of anti-diuretic hormone decreases so that you produce larger quantities of urine shortly after a float, contributing to the fall in BP.
* Because sensory deprivation in a floatation tank allows the brain to focus in on the body (homeostatic feedback), most people can learn to slow their heartbeat and blood pressure at will with a little practice.

✳ Increased levels of natural, heroin-like chemicals (endorphins and encephalins) are secreted in the brain during a float – these help relaxation and probably also explain the euphoria that many floaters feel.

In people with hypertension, even a single float lasting 45 minutes will lower BP. This effect continues gradually across repeated sessions and the lower blood pressure is maintained for several days after floatation therapy stops. As well as helping hypertension, floatation therapy lowers raised cholesterol levels, relieves chronic pain and reduces other unwanted effects of stress.

BIOFEEDBACK

Biofeedback is a visualization technique – usually practised during meditation or floatation therapy – in which adepts learn to control a body function that is not usually under voluntary control, such as speeding or slowing the heart rate at will.

Research in America suggests that 8 out of 10 people with hypertension can bring their blood pressure under control using a simple biofeedback method. This involves placing a thermometer on the floor, then putting your bare foot on top of it so your skin is in close contact with it. You then concentrate on your feet enough to raise their skin temperature to 36°C – use mental images of your foot resting on a hot water bottle, and imagine your feet getting warmer and warmer.

Biofeedback probably lowers BP by encouraging dilation of the peripheral circulation, including that in the skin, which opens up the circulation enough to let blood pressure fall.

YOGA

Yoga is an oriental technique that involves postural exercises, breathing techniques and relaxation. It is excellent for improving joint suppleness, relieving stress and reducing high blood pressure.

Suggested Lifestyle Changes for People with Hypertension

✳ If you smoke, try to stop – chemicals in cigarettes damage artery linings, cause spasm and constriction of vessels, and raise your blood pressure.
✳ Increase the amount of exercise you take – try to walk as much as possible, and use the stairs instead of the lift.
✳ Do not drink excessive amounts of alcohol, although moderate intakes seem to be protective.
✳ Watch your caffeine intake, especially if you are under stress.
✳ Lose any excess weight (*see Chapter 20*) – this can sometimes lower blood pressure enough to bring it back down to normal and get you off treatment.
✳ Eat a healthy diet with plenty of fresh fruit and vegetables for protective vitamins, minerals and fibre (*see Chapter 8*).
✳ Cut back on your salt intake by not adding it during cooking or at the table (*see Chapter 7*).

- If you are diabetic, make sure your blood sugar levels are well controlled.
- Try to avoid stressful situations and take time out to relax – stress hormones send BP rocketing.

  Try transcendental meditation, floatation therapy, biofeedback, yoga, or have an aromatherapy bath with oils of lavender, marjoram or ylang ylang.

 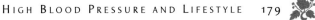

Useful Addresses

Please send a stamped, self-addressed envelope if writing
to an organization for information or a list of practitioners

British Heart Foundation
14 Fitzhardinge Street
London
W1H 4DH
Heart Health Line tel: 0870 600 6566
www.bhf.org.uk

British Dietetic Association
5th Floor
Charles House
148/9 Great Charles Street
Birmingham
B3 3HT
Tel: 0121 200 8080
www.bda.uk.com

The Nutrition Society
10 Cambridge Court
210 Shepherds Bush Road
London
W6 7NJ
Fax: 020 7602 1756
www.nutsoc.org.uk

British Association of Nutritional Therapists
27 Old Gloucester Street
London
WC1N 3XX
Send £2 plus a large (A4) SAE for a list of
therapists.

Institute for Optimum Nutrition
Blades Court
Deodar Road
London
SW15 2NU
Tel: 020 8877 9993
www.ion.ac.uk

The National Institute of Medical Herbalists
56 Longbrooke Street
Exeter
EX4 8HA
Tel: 01392 426022

General Council and Register of Naturopaths
Frazer House
6 Netherall Gardens
London
NW3 5RR
Tel: 020 7435 8728

Index